ADHD - From Etiology to Comorbidity

Edited by Hojka Gregorič Kumperščak

Published in London, United Kingdom

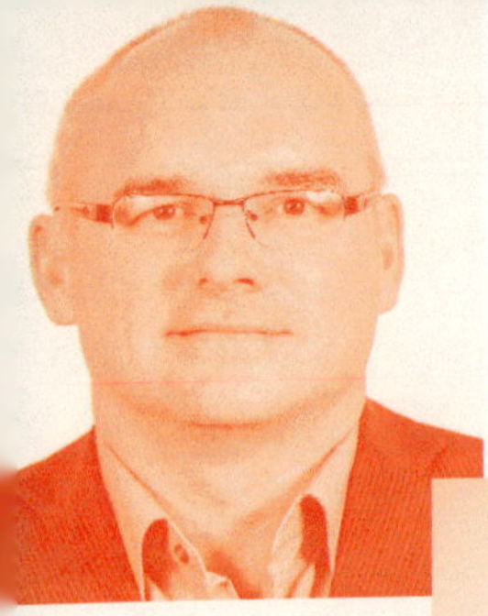
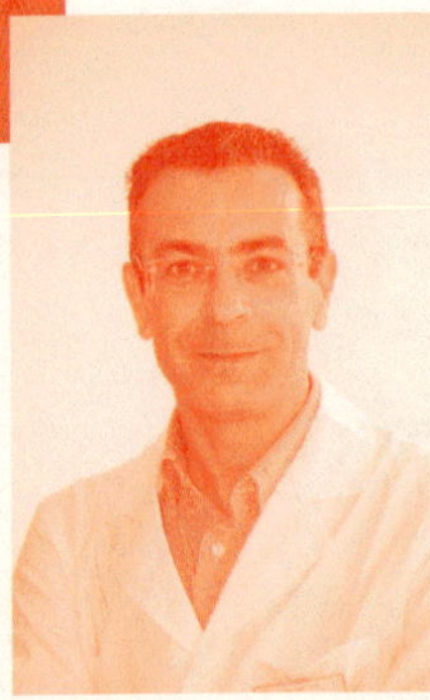
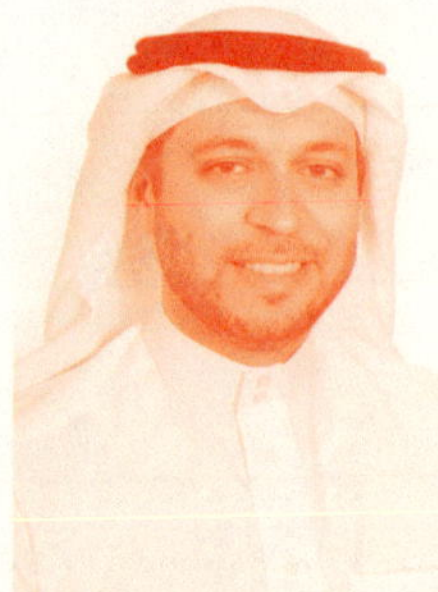
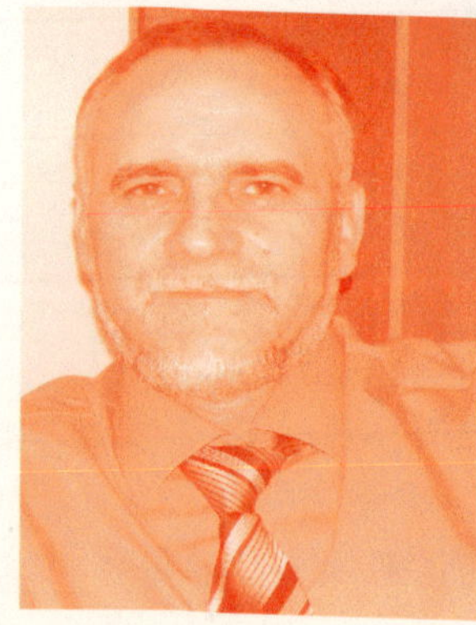
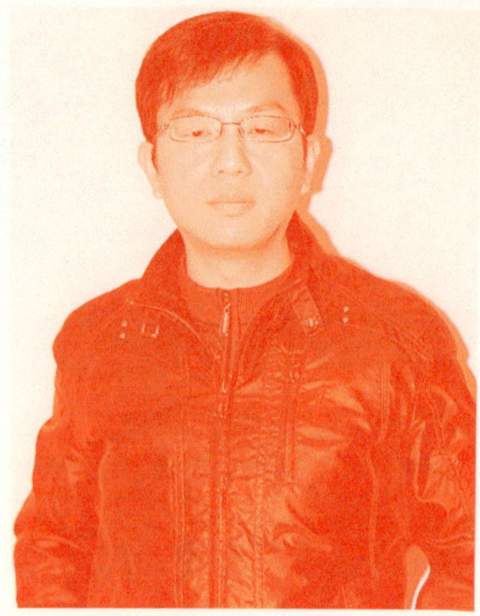
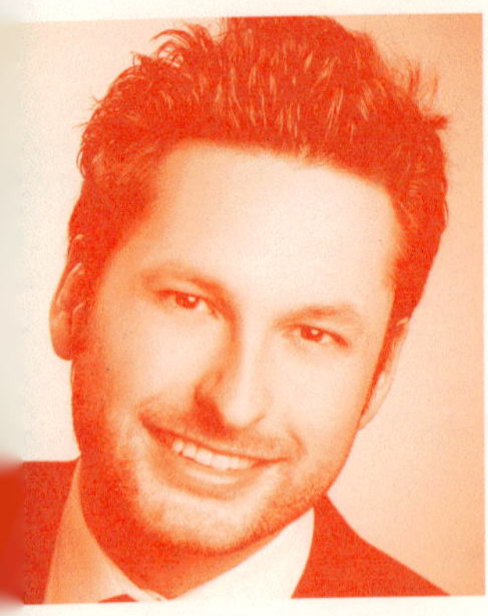
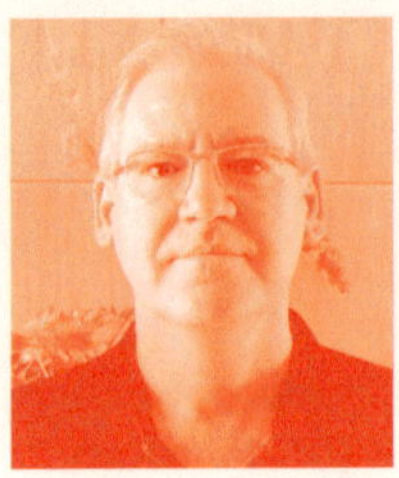

IntechOpen

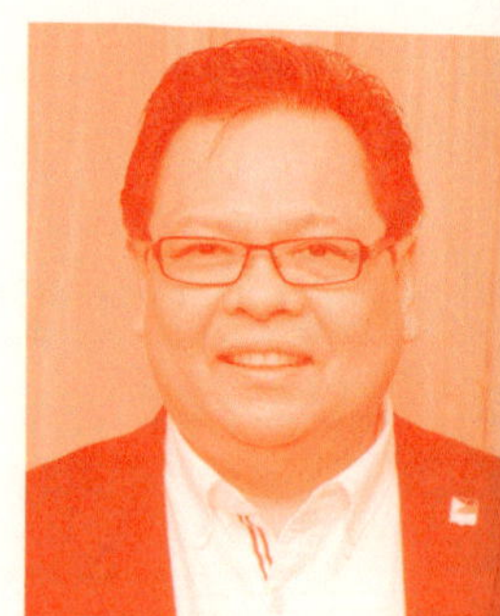
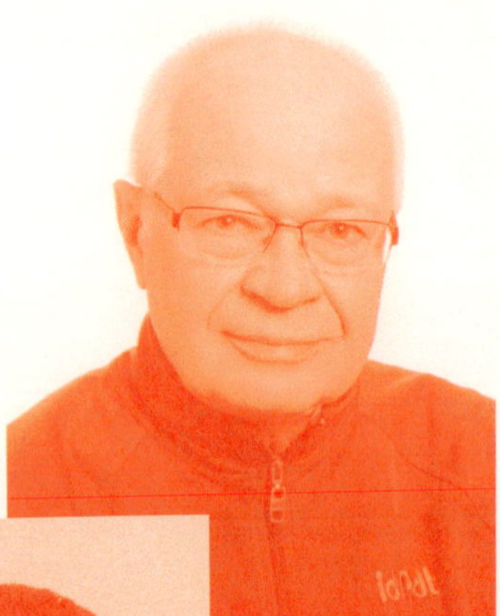
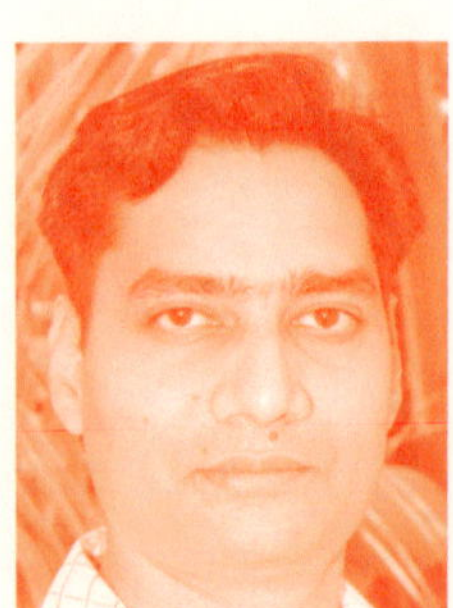
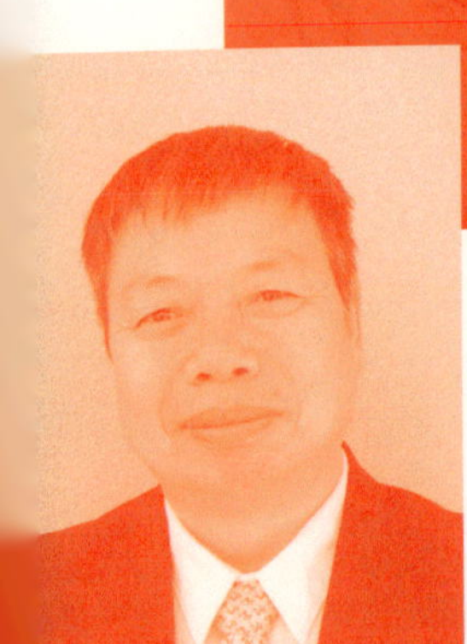
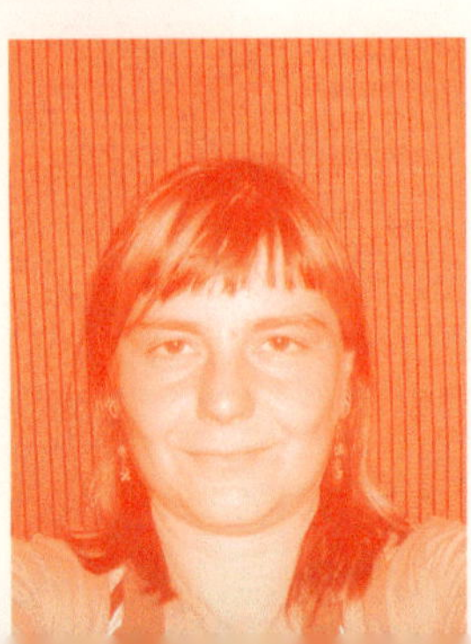
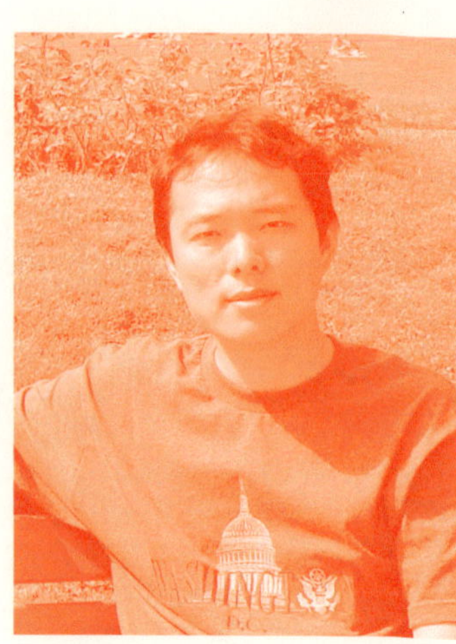

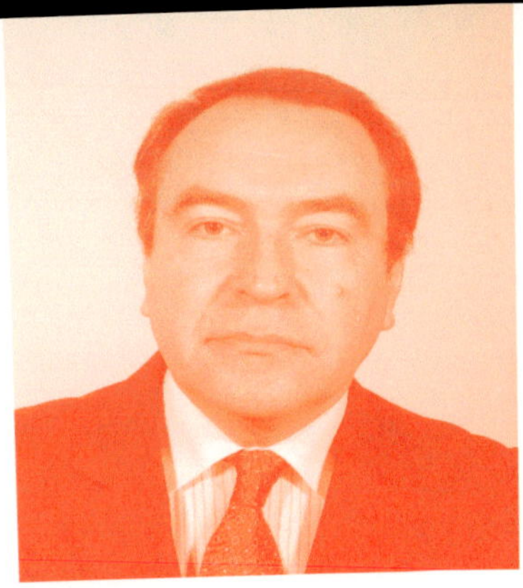
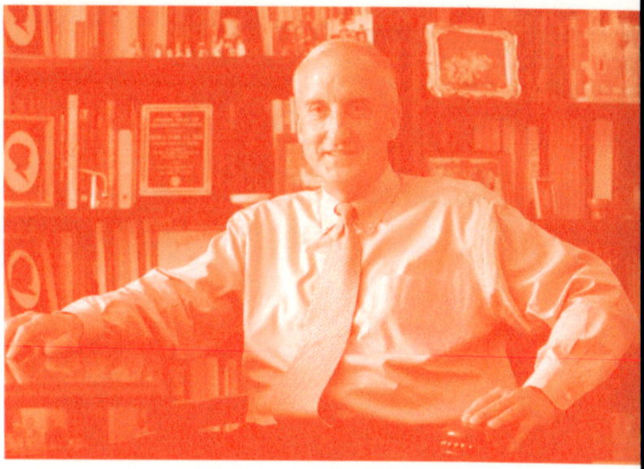
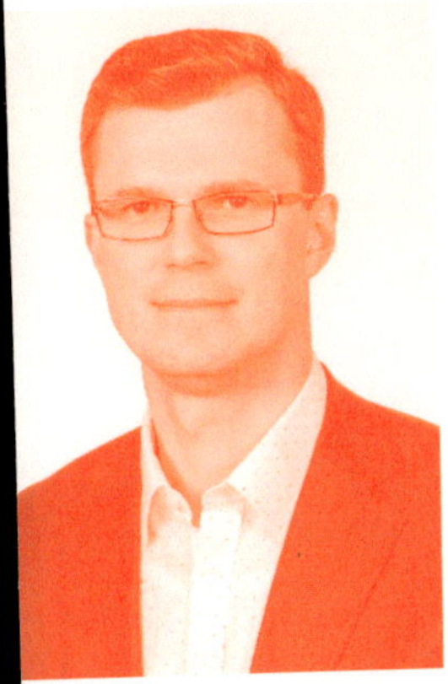
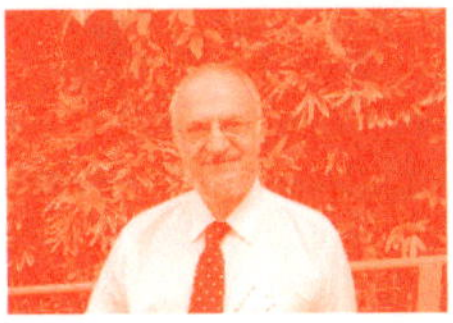
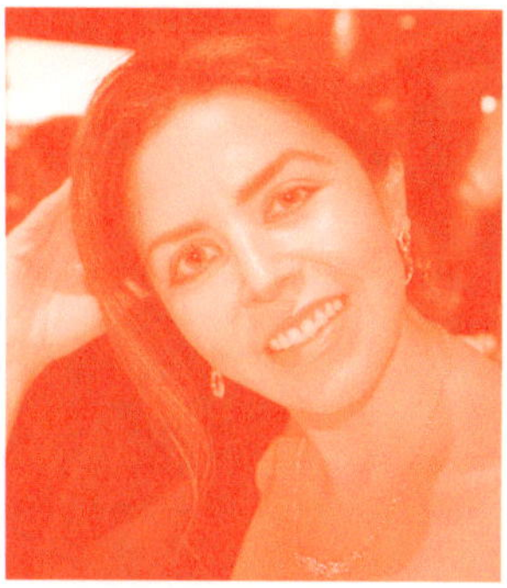

Supporting open minds since 2005

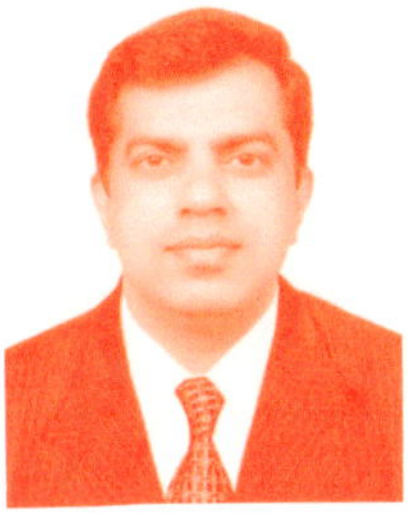
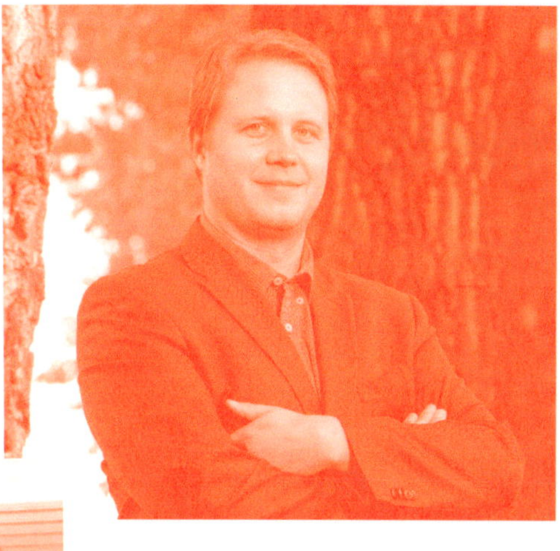
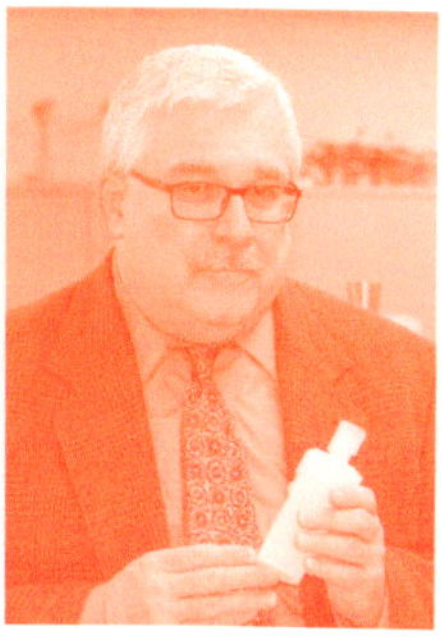
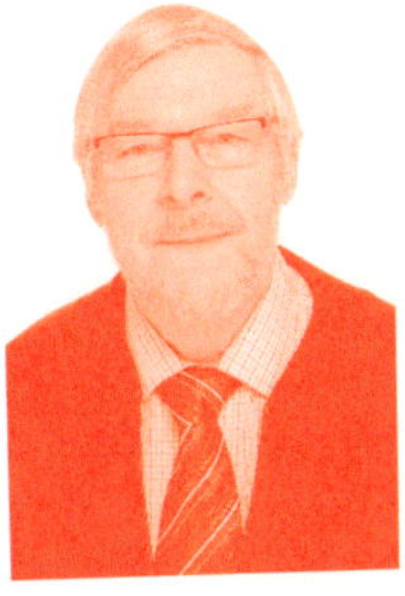
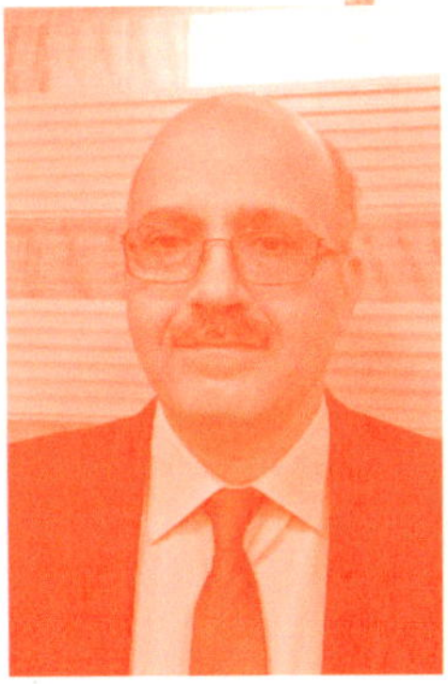
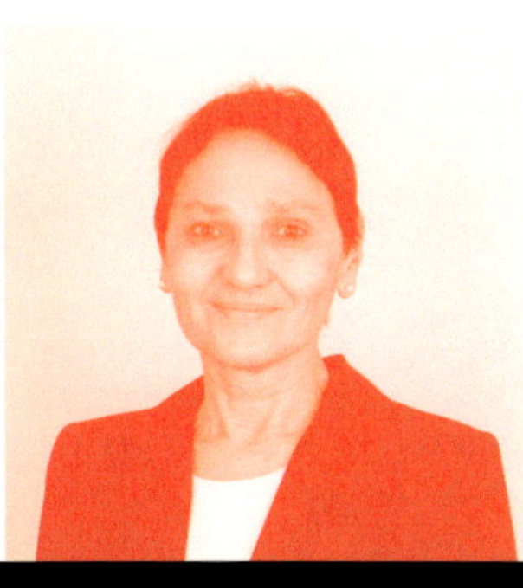
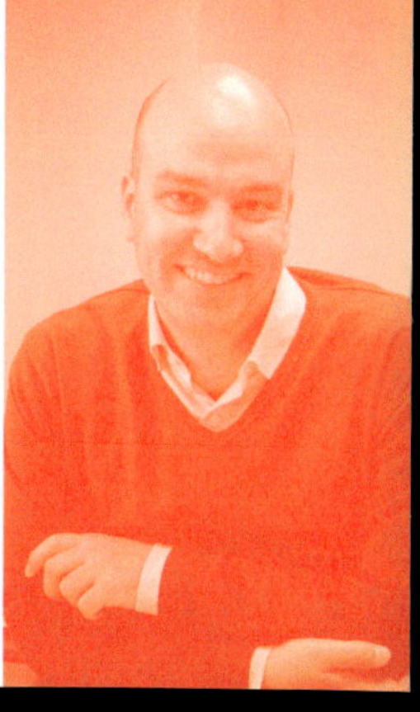

ADHD - From Etiology to Comorbidity
http://dx.doi.org/10.5772/intechopen.87283
Edited by Hojka Gregorič Kumperščak

Contributors
Hojka Gregoric Kumperscak, Clay Brites, Anja Plemenitaš Ilješ, Juan Carlos López, Annabel Jiménez-Soto, Juan Pedro Vargas, Estrella Díaz, Danijela Krgović, Marija Burgić Radmanović, Sanela Burgić

First published in London, United Kingdom, 2021 by IntechOpen
IntechOpen is the global imprint of INTECHOPEN LIMITED, registered in England and Wales, registration number: 11086078, 5 Princes Gate Court, London, SW7 2QJ, United Kingdom
Printed in Croatia

British Library Cataloguing-in-Publication Data
A catalogue record for this book is available from the British Library

Additional hard and PDF copies can be obtained from orders@intechopen.com

ADHD - From Etiology to Comorbidity
Edited by Hojka Gregorič Kumperščak
p. cm.
Print ISBN 978-1-83962-475-9
Online ISBN 978-1-83962-495-7
eBook (PDF) ISBN 978-1-83962-496-4

For EU product safety concerns:
IN TECH d.o.o., Prolaz Marije Krucifikse Kozulić 3, 51000 Rijeka, Croatia, info@intechopen.com or visit our website at intechopen.com.

Meet the editor

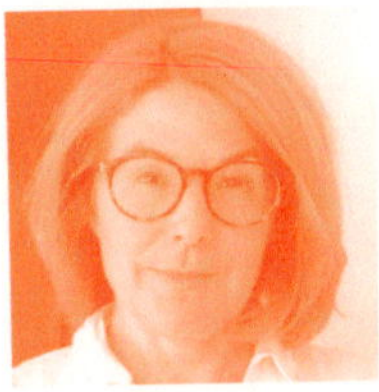

Assoc. Prof. Hojka Gregorič Kumperščak, MD, Ph.D., was born in Maribor, Slovenia in 1970. She finished the Faculty of Medicine in Ljubljana, Slovenia in 1996. She trained in child and adolescent psychiatry in Slovenia and abroad (Italy, UK, Germany, and Switzerland). She has served as chair of the Department of Psychiatry, Faculty of Medicine, University of Maribor, Slovenia, since January 2017, and has been head of the Child and Adolescent Psychiatry Unit, University Clinical Center, Maribor, since 2008. She is the president of the Slovenian Association for Child and Adolescent Psychiatry. She is also the national coordinator–training director for Child and Adolescent Psychiatry in Slovenia and secretary of the Child and Adolescent section of the Union European Medical Specialists (UEMS-CAP). She is a member of the editorial board for the World Psychiatric Association's journal, Child and Adolescent Psychiatry. Her clinical work is mainly with adolescents with personality and psychotic disorders. Her research work focuses on the genetics of developmental disorders including ADHD and early-onset schizophrenia. Dr. Kumperščak is an adolescent identity treatment psychotherapist and trainer. She has written many scientific articles and book chapters on different CAP topics.

Contents

Preface

Attention Deficit Hyperactivity Disorder (ADHD) is not only the most prevalent neurodevelopmental disorder but also a very contradictory one. This book provides a comprehensive overview of ADHD, with a focus on diagnosis and comorbidity.

The Introductory Chapter, "ADHD Has Many Faces" by Prof. Hojka Gregoric Kumperscak, presents ADHD as a disorder with a vivid history of changing names, diagnostic criteria, and clinical point of view. Previously, it was considered a disorder that affected children only. Recently, however, there is no doubt that ADHD can affect adults as well, but with different clinical presentation. Thus, it is critical to understand how the clinical picture of the disorder changes with development.

Chapter 2, "Traditional Scales Diagnosis and Endophenotypes in Attentional Deficits Disorders: Are We on the Right Track?" by Annabel Jiménez-Soto, Juan Pedro Vargas, Estrella Díaz and Juan Carlos López, discusses the necessity of broadening diagnostic thinking away from the boundaries of traditional assessment (based on questionnaires and behavioural scales). One way to do this is to study the vulnerable traits associated with impulsivity and attentional deficit. In a quantitative fashion, these traits could be used to define a specific endophenotype. This view would allow a more precise medical/psychological assessment of the patient along the life span, avoiding a diagnosis based on the number of symptoms only.

When working with parents it is important to determine whether there is a genetic basis for ADHD. New genetic studies bring deeper and more concise knowledge about the disorder's aetiology. As discussed in Chapter 3, "Role of Copy Number Variations in ADHD" by Danijela Krgović, copy number variations (CNVs) have an important role in the aetiology of neurodevelopmental disorders (NDDs), including ADHD. CNVs provide new opportunities for studying and managing psychiatric disorders in general. Identification of disease-associated genes and knowledge of their molecular functions will lead to a better understanding of their disease pathology and hopefully enable better diagnosis and treatment. Genetic counselling for polygenic disorders with complex genetic architecture like ADHD is challenging due to variable phenotypic outcomes and incomplete penetrance encountered in most genetic disorders. Therefore, understanding molecular aetiology is useful for patient management in terms of improving risk predictions, screening for extra-psychiatric features, and tailoring treatment to the individual.

Comorbidity is a rule, especially if ADHD is not recognised and treated early. As discussed in Chapter 4, "Comorbidity in Children and Adolescents with ADHD" the presence of comorbidities largely depends on case definition, assessment methodology, and control group. Studies show that 67%–80% of children diagnosed with ADHD have at least one other diagnosis, and almost half of them have two. Two-thirds of children with ADHD have at least one other psychiatric disorder. Specific learning difficulties are more common in people with ADHD than in the general population with a prevalence of 45%. The most common learning difficulties in children with ADHD are in the areas of reading, spelling, writing, and math.

Children with ADHD have greater learning difficulties than children who have only specific learning difficulties.

It is crucial to be aware of comorbidities because they complicate the diagnostic and therapeutic processes as well as affect the course and prognosis of the disorder. Assessment and support in comorbid disorders are often as important as the assessment and treatment of ADHD symptoms.

Chapter 5, "ADHD and Impact on Language" by Clay Brites, discusses language abnormalities as some of the most common ADHD comorbidities. The language problem in ADHD can be expressed at any age and at different intensity levels. These abnormalities can negatively affect daily activities and the learning process, which depends on proper language acquisition during the child's development. The abnormalities in language result in greater unsatisfactory evolution and many problems in verbal and non-verbal abilities, adversely impacting academic life because of losses in reading and writing appropriation. Thus, it is essential to understand the facts that interrelate ADHD with the cognitive and language development process and where and how ADHD neurobiological dysfunctions affect the dynamic of the neural network responsible for receptive, integrative, and expressive language structure at different child neurodevelopment levels.

Chapter 6, "Adult Attention-Deficit/Hyperactivity Disorder and Substance Use Disorder: A Systematic Review of the Literature" by Anja Plemenitaš Ilješ, discusses untreated ADHD and how it is highly comorbid with substance use disorder (SUD). ADHD is diagnosed in up to 20% of patients with SUD. The two disorders are believed to have shared pathophysiology. ADHD is associated with most dependence diagnoses. Evidence on pharmacological treatment is limited, but new trials support the use of a higher dose of long-acting stimulants combined with psychotherapy. The decision to treat adult ADHD in the context of SUD depends on various factors, so clinical decisions should be individualized and based on a careful analysis of the advantages and disadvantages of pharmacological treatment for ADHD in the context of SUD.

This book addresses all these issues to bring more clarity and understanding of ADHD to clinicians, scientists, researchers, and family members of those with the disorder.

Hojka Gregorič Kumperščak
Department of Paediatrics and University of Maribor,
Faculty of Medicine,
University Medical Centre Maribor,
Maribor, Slovenia

Section 1

New Approaches in ADHD Diagnostic

Chapter 1

Introductory Chapter: ADHD Has Many Faces

Hojka Gregoric Kumperscak

1. Introduction

Attention deficit hyperactivity disorder (ADHD) is nowadays not only the most prevalent neurodevelopmental disorder [1] but also the most troublesome mental disorder that I have come across. A problem arises already with the name. International Classification of Diseases (ICD-10) uses the term Hyperkinetic Disorder [2] whereas as per the Diagnostic and Statistical Manual of Mental Disorders (DSM-5), the term is ADHD [3]. This is not only a semantic problem but the diagnosis criteria are significantly different (DSM has broader and less strict diagnosis criteria, so it encompasses more people) and lead to substantial differences in both its prevalence and treatment [4].

Not so long ago, students at medical faculties were taught that ADHD was a children's disorder that abated during adolescence and was non-existent in adulthood. Today, both clinical experience and all of the studies show that, in the majority, the disorder persists into adulthood but manifests itself differently.

2. From symptoms to broader diagnostic thinking

The most recognisable symptom group of ADHD is hyperactivity that is only seen in childhood. It does not take much knowledge to think of ADHD in a child that moves, runs and climbs incessantly, regardless of the dangers, and of that child being hyperactive. The problem of recognising ADHD in a child is already posed by clinical presentation without hyperactivity (ADD).

Although most children with ADHD have hyperactivity, it already abates in adolescence. It gets replaced by an inner restlessness. Again, we find ourselves in front of a major differential diagnostic problem. Which adolescent is not internally restless or tense? The developmental tasks that adolescents face lead to inner restlessness in at least some developmental periods in almost all of them. Inner restlessness is also a common complaint of adolescents and adults with depression, anxiety, psychosis or other mental disorders. Few experts think first of ADHD in case of inner restlessness.

Another group of ADHD symptoms is equally 'problematic'–impulsiveness. Impulsiveness is also a norm in adolescents since youth is essentially a synonym for quick, reckless decisions–jumping over a ditch where there is a bridge. Impulsiveness is also characteristic of many other mental disorders apart from ADHD. It is at the heart of behavioural disorders, some personality, organic and other mental disorders. The problem with recognising ADHD is its varied symptoms shared with so many other mental disorders or life periods. Which expert would think first of ADHD upon hearing complaints of inner restlessness and impulsiveness in adolescents or adults?

IntechOpen

For this reason, it is necessary to broaden the diagnostic thinking out of the boundaries of traditional assessment (based on questionnaires and behavioural scales) in work with patients and parents and diagnostic in general. When working with parents, it is good to know how hereditary the disease is and how important the etiological factor genetic is (around 75%) [1, 5]. It is necessary to know the influence of genetics and think of endophenotypes. The study of vulnerable traits associated with impulsiveness and attention deficit provides for an alternative diagnostic approach. Quantitatively, these traits could define a specific endophenotype. This view would allow for a more precise medical/psychological assessment focus on the patient along their lifespan, avoiding diagnosis based on the number of symptoms [6–8].

3. ADHD can be a devastating disorder if not recognised and treated in childhood

Children with ADHD usually stand out with their behaviour featuring hyperactivity and impulsiveness. Many also have comorbid language difficulties and other learning disorders, often resulting in academic underachievement. For this reason, these children find themselves more quickly, more frequently and more intensively subjected to criticism by teachers, parents and peers. Children with ADHD are more likely to be socially excluded by their peers than children without ADHD. The nature of ADHD makes it harder for children to concentrate and follow the playing rules, forcing them to react too quickly and inappropriately. Children with ADHD can do extremely well in individual sports (swimming, cycling, running), but they do not do well in team sports, sooner or later, they come into conflict with their teammates/coaches/referees precisely because of the characteristics described above. They develop a poor self-image, begin to withdraw from society, and may become anxious, depressed or behaviourally problematic. They are more likely than the general population to seek reassurance from alcohol and psychoactive substances (PAS), using them as a form of self-medication. Thus, secondary problems, difficulties and mental disorders become superimposed on the 'pure clinical picture of ADHD' as the child develops. Less studied, although also important, is the effect of ADHD on language. A 'pure' clinical presentation is no longer seen in adolescents with ADHD. It is hidden in depression/dysphoria/irritability, PAS abuse, anxiety, poor self-image and behavioural disorder. It is only when (if) all these layers are slowly peeled away that we get to the core problem—ADHD.

In adults, there is another problem: ADHD symptoms become internalised. If someone has always been forgetful, deviant, unpunctual, conflicting, then one adopts these symptoms as personality traits rather than symptoms of a disorder that could be treated. This is also how others see them—as distracted, unreliable, rarely finish what they start—not as someone with a mental disorder. Thus, in adults, the problem of ADHD continues into treatment. Even when we have diagnosed ADHD in an adult, it is difficult to motivate them to seek treatment. They ask questions like: if they have been like this since birth, are we going to change their personality with treatment? It takes a lot of education and motivation to get them to accept and persevere with treatment. It is necessary to explain that treatment will enable them to express all the creative and positive things that have not yet come out. It will allow them to concentrate on important things rather than running from one thing to another and finally completing only a few or none of the tasks. Their interpersonal relationships will also change for the better, as they will be able to listen to others and not react so impulsively without any consideration of the consequences.

4. ADHD: is there anything positive?

We should not forget about the possible positive consequences of ADHD—high energy, the ability to react quickly, the ability to multitask, to have innovative ideas, not to stick to routines, and to find new solutions. The list goes on and on. It is said that a person with ADHD had an evolutionary advantage in the past. In the wild, it was vital to be able to pay attention to several stimuli at the same time, to react to any one of them quickly and without thinking about the consequences. Unfortunately, today's high-performance and efficiency-oriented times are not favourable to people with ADHD. Today's times demand good concentration on a single problem, completion of tasks on time, punctuality, precision, the ability to sit through even the most tedious learning/working task, thoughtful reactions and predictable solutions. Nowadays, even 6-year-olds have to sit for 45 minutes at school, which is very questionable from a developmental point of view. Therein lies the answer to the question of how it is that we are diagnosing this disorder increasingly frequently. We are detecting it more because nowadays, people with it are significantly less able to function on a daily basis than they were a few decades ago. If we know that hyperactivity is a symptom of ADHD that abates first, it is understandable that children entering the school at 7/8 years of age did not have the same problems as today's younger first graders. In the not-so-distant past, children were free after school or involved in significantly fewer after-school activities than today, and their potential attention deficit disorder did not have so much 'space' to become a problem. The movement used to be something natural and given to all children, but today we find that children are physically incapable. It is not the present time that has made ADHD, but in today's time, people with ADHD, who are no more numerous than in the past, are simply decompensating sooner.

Author details

Hojka Gregoric Kumperscak[1,2]

1 Child and Adolescent Psychiatry Unit, University Medical Centre Maribor, Maribor, Slovenia

2 Faculty of Medicine, University of Maribor, Maribor, Slovenia

*Address all correspondence to: hojka.gregoric@guest.arnes.si

References

[1] Polanczyk G, de Lima MS, Horta BL, Biederman J, Rohde LA. The worldwide prevalence of ADHD: A systematic review and metaregression analysis. The American Journal of Psychiatry. 2007;**164**:942-948

[2] World Health Organization. International Statistical Classification of Diseases and Related Health Problems (ICD-10). 10th Revision ed. World Health Organization; 2010

[3] American Psychiatric Association. *Diagnostic and Statistical Manual of Mental Disorders*. 5th ed. Arlington, VA: American Psychiatric Publishing; 2013

[4] Taylor E, Döpfner M, Sergeant J, Asherson P, Banaschewski T, Buitelaar J, et al. European clinical guidelines for hyperkinetic disorder - First upgrade. European Child & Adolescent Psychiatry. 2004;(Suppl 13):17-30

[5] Van Loo KM, Martens GJ. Genetic and environmental factors in complex neurodevelopmental disorders. Current Genomics. 2007;**8**:429-444

[6] Miranda P, Cox CD, Alexander M, Danev S, Lakey JRT. In quest of pathognomonic/endophenotypic markers of Attention Deficit Hyperactivity Disorder (ADHD): Potential of EEG-based frequency analysis and ERPs to better detect, prevent and manage ADHD. Med Devices (Auckl). 2020;**13**:115-137. DOI: 10.2147/mder.S241205

[7] Slaats-Willemse D, Swaab-Barneveld H, De Sonneville L, Van Der Meulen E, Buitelaar J. Deficient response inhibition as a cognitive endophenotype of ADHD. Journal of the American Academy of Child and Adolescent Psychiatry. 2003;**42**(10): 1242-1248. DOI: 10.1097/00004583-200310000-00016

[8] Vargas JP, Díaz E, Portavella M, López JC. Animal models of maladaptive traits: Disorders in sensorimotor gating and attentional quantifiable responses as possible endophenotypes. Frontiers in Psychology. 2016;7(206):1-9. DOI: 10.3389/fpsyg.2016.00206

Chapter 2

Traditional Scales Diagnosis and Endophenotypes in Attentional Deficits Disorders: Are We on the Right Track?

Annabel Jiménez-Soto, Juan Pedro Vargas, Estrella Díaz and Juan Carlos López

Abstract

The concept of ADHD has changed widely through the history of mental health classification manuals. In the past three decades, the number of ADHD diagnoses has hugely increased worldwide. One of the reasons to explain this fact could be the lack of precision, differentiation and adjust of the criteria and indicators of this disease. Research has detected as well, some subjectivity bias in the traditional assessment (based in questionnaires and behavioral scales), which is affecting to the precision in the diagnose and to the further adjustment to the treatment. In this regard, these diagnoses are based in symptoms but not in etiology of the disorder. Therefore, different disorders will share the same treatment, regardless etiology. A different approach is based on the study of vulnerable traits associated with impulsivity and attentional deficit. In a quantitative fashion; these traits could be used to define a specific endophenotype. This view would allow us a more precise medical/psychological assessment focus on patient along the life spam, avoiding a diagnostic based on the number of symptoms. Here, we discuss about the differences between traditional diagnosis scales and the possibilities to find endophenotypes in order to address a specific treatment.

Keywords: ADHD, assessment, diagnosis, impulsivity, endophenotypes

1. Introduction

Attention Deficit Hyperactivity Disorder, better known as ADHD, is one of the most common diagnoses among children nowadays and its prevalence worldwide is estimated at 5% for children, and 2.5% for adults [1]. However, the prevalence showed in different studies and countries varies quite a lot and does so in wide ranges, which is commonly associated with theoretical and methodological approaches to understand and assess the disorder. Understood as a brain disorder, ADHD has been defined on multiple occasions trying to account for the symptom variability and heterogeneity present in people with ADHD [2–5]. Due to the great symptomatic variability showed by these patients, the lack of biological or genetic markers of the disorder recognized by the APA itself and the heterogeneity expressed in the cognitive functioning of these individuals [1], explanatory models of the disease are increasingly abundant and diverse, making the diagnose a complicated, questioned and commonly criticized process.

There are different times in the history of medicine, psychology and psychiatry in which several authors identified ADHD as a syndrome for the first time [6–8], even though it is not until 1968 when the disorder was full described in one of the main manuals of mental health [9]. In its second edition, the diagnostic category for childhood and adolescence included a new syndrome that was termed as "hyperkinetic reaction". The manual described this syndrome as a disorder characterized by overactivity behavior, restlessness, easy distraction and short attention span. It was more common in children and generally improved during adolescence [9]. Afterwards, the DSM III published for the first time a reference to the disorder as we know it currently. Named as "attention deficit disorder" and included into the behavioral category of diseases that occurs in the infancy or childhood, the diagnosis was subdivided into two subtypes: attention deficit hyperactivity disorder and attention deficit non-hyperactivity disorder. On the one hand, it is mentioned among the clarifications that the symptoms may not be directly observable by the clinician [10]. In addition, it included indicators among the criteria of the disorder such as "often does not seem to listen" or "often acts before thinking", constructs that are hardly observable in an objective way.

In 1987, the American Psychiatric Association revised the text of the third manual that resulted in the DSM III-R. This review included ADHD as a discrete disorder, for which it was necessary to display both related symptoms, inattention and hyperactivity. If just inattention symptoms were present, but not the hyperactivity, the diagnosis was "undifferentiated attention deficit disorder" [11]. Despite the increased requirements for the diagnosis, the number of people being diagnosed kept growing. A few years after the fourth version of the diagnostic manual of mental disorders, published in 1994, described the basis of what we currently understand by ADHD. The disorder described affected three main axes: attention, hyperactivity and impulsivity. And it gave rise to different subtypes of the disorder that were classified into inattentive, hyperactive–impulsive, or combined [12]. Although it has been more than twenty years since this description, it is remarkable that an exhaustive differentiation between hyperactivity and impulsivity as constructs has not been made yet when ADHD is defined or assessed. Since then and until the last release of the Diagnostic Manual of Mental Disorders, there were no remarkable changes in the way of defining the disorder [13]. In contrast, the latest version of the manual, DSM 5 [1], makes some important changes in the disorder definition, its causes and specific characteristics. In this edition of the manual, ADHD is defined as a neurodevelopmental disorder, and in an inconsistent way, the age of symptoms onset was increased from seven to twelve years old. This change in the age of symptoms onset also applies to the ICD-11 versus ICD-10 versions [14, 15]. Furthermore, one of the most significant changes in DSM 5 for ADHD comes from the introduction of a paragraph that states: "The signs of the disorder may be minimal or absent when the individual receives frequent rewards for appropriate behavior, is under close supervision, in a new situation, participating in especially interesting activities, has constant external stimulation (e.g., with electronic displays), or is in situations where he or she interacts face-to-face with another person (e.g., in the clinician's office)" [1]. What could that possibly mean? We do not know what is the meaning of this statement, but the result of DSM 5 changes is a sharply increased prevalence of the disorder. This has gone hand in hand with modifications in the DSM, since diagnostic criteria in the recent version remain vague. That is the reason why nowadays is easier to receive a diagnosis based on these criteria than twenty years ago. DMS 5 relativizes the importance of symptoms, which goes from assuming "clear evidence of clinically significant dysfunction in the social, academic or occupational sphere" [13] to "interfering with or reducing the quality of life of any of them" [1]. In addition, the number of symptoms needed to meet the criteria for inattention or hyperactivity-impulsivity was reduced from six to five for adolescents and adults over 17 years old.

2. ADHD traditional assessment: what could be wrong?

Nowadays, the most used instruments to assess ADHD are tests and scales of behavior, which are usually completed by parents and teachers. These tools are generally based on the diagnostic indicators of ADHD, describing some symptoms or behavior included in the disorder. Although behavior scales and tests currently remain the most widely used assessment method, the validity and reliability of these tools are not consistent in the literature [16]. Even when clinical practice guidelines on ADHD have recommended a neuropsychological assessment of symptoms, beyond the subjective reports provided by scales and tests, at present, this assessment is still considered dispensable to establish the diagnosis of ADHD [16–19]. Fortunately, the use of neuropsychological tests to assess the effects of these patients is becoming increasingly common.

Perhaps one of the most important problems when assessing ADHD is the bias produced by the use of tests and behavioral scales. The subjective experience of responding to a survey can record biases such as social desirability, the anticipation of the hypothesis, and even false and premeditated responses. In addition, when relatives are the ones who report on the behavior of a third party, the problems of subjectivity are even greater [20]. This fact has been repeated for more than thirty years. Parents and teachers tend to rate up to 50% of healthy children as inattentive, distracted, restless or hyperactive [21]. This subjectivity is also sensitive to the halo effect, which has shown a bilateral effect between inattention and hyperactivity-impulsivity symptoms. That is, the greater the number of symptoms in one of the criteria, the higher the score in the other [22]. Moreover, depending on whether it is the mother, father or teacher who fill in the questionnaires, patients can be diagnosed with one or another subtype of the disorder [23], with parents reporting the most symptoms [24]. Besides, the correlation between parents and teachers' reports is generally low [25].

Another assessment problem about ADHD is related to development. That is, evaluation and diagnosis do not take into account that the symptoms of the disorder are not stable during the life span [26]. Additionally, according to the scientific literature, the persistence of the disorder in adulthood varies between 4 and 66% [27]. These diagnostic differences between youths and adults are usually explained by the existence of undiagnosable subthreshold ADHD in adults [28], or the existence of two syndromes with different trajectories [29]. In this regard, a recent study that followed a sample of people diagnosed with ADHD for nine years found that when the participants were 18 years old on average, only 16.7% still met the criteria for the diagnosis of ADHD, and 11% were classified as having sub-threshold ADHD [30]. This means that 72.3% of the whole sample did not show any disturbance after nine years of follow-up.

The fact that the symptoms are not stable over time is something we have known for over two decades now [26]. Nevertheless, the diagnostic criteria and indicators are the same for all age groups. The only difference we can find is related to the number of indicators needed to meet the criteria, where adults need five instead of six indicators to meet the criteria of inattention or hyperactivity-impulsivity. Something similar happens concerning symptoms shown in people with ADHD.

Despite the efforts to find functional subtypes within the disorder, findings have displayed a high diversity/heterogeneity in the symptoms and disturbances of the disorder [31, 32], that resembles the behavioral repertoire of these individuals [33]. This fact makes extremely difficult to accept the definition of the disorder as it is currently understood.

2.1 Comorbidity gets worse the current ADHD definition

Another great problem reported is the wide and diverse comorbidity commonly found in the disorder, such as the concurrent presence of a dissocial disorder or oppositional defiant disorder [34]. The problem is even greater if we consider that the three main axes of the disorder (hyperactivity, impulsivity and inattention) are affected in a wide variety of psychopathological conditions [35]. According to the DSM 5, there are up to 16 comorbidities frequently associated with the disorder, such as oppositional defiant disorder, autism spectrum disorders, anxiety, depression, intellectual disability, or other neurodevelopmental disorders [1]. They have also been assessed for their concurrent occurrence with ADHD, coordination disorders, substance abuse disorders and even Tourette's syndrome [35].

Several authors have suggested that comorbidities are variable because they are specifically related to each subtype of the disorder. Thus, externalizing problems seem to be more comorbid in patients with hyperactive–impulsive or combined subtype, while internalizing is more common in people with inattentive subtype [36]. According to APA, ADHD combined subtype is associated with the oppositional defiant disorder in approximately 50% of the diagnosed cases and up to 25% of the inattentive subtype, whereas behavioral disorders among all the diagnoses are present in a quarter of them [1].

In this regard, people with ADHD generally display more symptoms associated with anxiety disorders or depression than general population, and these comorbid symptoms are also stable over time [37]. Concerning depression, a meta-analysis with more than 300,000 participants reported that ADHD was also comorbidly related to the occurrence of suicidal behavior [38]. These facts make that pure diagnosis of ADHD cases are very rare and complicated to find [35]. For instance, a study analyzed 1919 cases of diagnosed ADHD, finding that 66% of participants had at least one comorbidity with learning, sleep, anxiety or opposition disorders [39]. The overlap of symptoms in ADHD and other disorders is a quite important problem in the assessment, and it represents a challenge for its correct diagnosis [40]. This could be the reason why diagnostic criteria and indicators of the DSM 5 show a lack of validity. It is difficult to think of a child who is not "hard to keep up with" or "runs or talks too much." That is, many times the symptoms described for ADHD define the usual and normal behavior of children [33].

We tried to assess how people interpret the measure of ADHD symptoms in a survey made by our laboratory. Using the diagnostic criteria to explore the symptoms of ADHD among the general population, participants indicate as present in their behavioral repertoire on average at least five symptoms of the disorder, being more frequent the symptoms of inattention than those of hyperactivity/impulsivity [41]. With these indicators, many children who do not suffer from this disorder, but show some behavior outside of what is considered "normal", could easily be diagnosed with ADHD if just the DSM's criteria were used to assess the disorder. Thus, the current overdiagnosis might be due, among other problems, to the lack of consensus in the evaluation criteria [42]. For some authors, this fact makes DSM not to be reliable enough for ADHD diagnosis [33], and therefore other criteria should be considered for an accurate ADHD diagnostic [43].

It might appear that symptoms described in the indicators of ADHD usually define the normal behavior of children [33]. This explains why the criteria for maintenance of the symptoms in time and the contexts in which they appear are so important to evaluate when assessing this disorder. Currently if a child presents some behavior related to the description of ADHD, it is more than likely that he or she will receive the diagnosis. Although DSM 5 and ICD 11 focus on specific situations and how long a symptom lasts, the environmental triggers are not usually assessed, addressing the assessing to behavior patient. What is most disturbing is the fact that diagnosis is also defined in light of these described behavior, which would lead to a problem of reification pointed out by several authors [44–46].

2.2 Hyperactivity and impulsivity: different concepts, same diagnose

Another problem of criteria and indicators is related to hyperactivity and impulsivity concepts. Although both are defined in the DSM with different indicators for the disorder (6 for hyperactivity and 3 for impulsivity), they share the diagnostic category of hyperactive–impulsive [1], giving rise to a single subtype of the disorder. However, we currently know that hyperactivity and impulsivity belong to different constructs and domains and they are not understood as parts of a continuum.

Impulsivity is defined as a multidimensional concept, and it includes problems in decision making processes regarding long/short term reinforcement, a lack of behavioral inhibition related to future consequences, and an inappropriate behavior [2, 47, 48]. In addition, impulsive behavior displays a lack of sensitivity to negative consequences, and fast and unplanned responses [49]. Thus, impulsive behavior is a kind of no reflective behavior defined as a failure in inhibitory processes. This might be due to lower development of executive functions, getting worse in specific context as familiar or academic situations [50, 51]. It is commonly agreed that an impulsive person is one who "usually speaks or acts without reflection or caution, allowing himself or herself to be carried away by the impression of the moment". In contrast, we define hyperactivity as a "behavior characterized by excess activity".

Although both are expressed through lack of control, impulsivity could be better understood as a lack of cognitive inhibition and hyperactivity as a lack of motor inhibition. To verify this, some authors have evaluated the levels of hyperactivity and impulsivity in a sample of more than 10,000 healthy children, concluding emphatically that the measures of hyperactivity and impulsivity address different constructs [52]. In this regard, it is not complicated to imagine a person of any age who can be very energetic, in terms of activity, and yet be extremely reflective in terms of decision making. In the same way, we can also imagine someone who is not very energetic in his or her daily activities and notwithstanding is very impulsive when it comes to decision making. In light of all these results, we can see that the assessment of ADHD is a rather complicated process. There are no specific diagnostic tests to assess the disorder objectively, and the current assessment process is not free of problems and biases, which makes diagnosis even more difficult. The assessment of ADHD cannot and should not be carried out exclusively using questionnaire reports and behavior scales [53]. Only the combined use of reports and neuropsychological tests would produce an adequate assessment of the disorder [54], since the scales and tests do not measure the same as the experimental tasks [55].

2.3 ADHD treatment: do all roads lead to Rome?

According to DSM 5, a diagnosis of ADHD can lead to three different subtypes of the disorder: predominantly inattentive, the criteria of inattention is met, but not those of hyperactivity-impulsivity; predominantly hyperactive–impulsive, the criteria of hyperactivity-impulsivity are met, but not those of inattention; and the third subtype would be a combined presentation of the disorder, where both traits of inattention and hyperactivity-impulsivity would be affected [1]. In addition, the manual also includes two diagnostic categories when the criteria for the main subtypes are not met: other specified attention-deficit/hyperactivity disorder and unspecified attention-deficit/hyperactivity disorder. Nevertheless, there are no main differences in the therapeutical interventions and psychopharmacological treatments for these ADHD subtypes, and all of them will probably receive the same health/medical cares.

ADHD is usually treated as a problem of neurochemical dysfunction, accordingly the treatment commonly used is the administration of psychostimulants, which in a high number of cases reduces the frequency and duration of symptoms [17]. That is, regardless of the subtype diagnosed, patients are usually treated, at least in the initial phase, with the same drug. However, we now know that, although the systemic administration of stimulants such as methylphenidate, a psychostimulant that acts by inhibiting the reuptake of dopamine and noradrenaline, improves the symptoms for a while in most cases, but not in the long term [56]. This situation causes the beginning of continuous changes in treatments. This fact clearly indicates that the problems associated with this disorder depend on several pathways. One of them seems to be dependent on prefrontal dopaminergic pathways, and at the other extreme, we can find the opposite profile, triggering a pattern probably independent on these prefrontal pathways. In any case, at present we do not have diagnostic tools that allow us to identify these different populations within the same diagnosis [41].

2.4 ADHD as a neurodevelopmental problem: is it possible to find an anatomical profile?

Although the ADHD is considered as a neurodevelopmental disorder, in the last years there is an increasing number of studies that point to the possibility that ADHD can emerge in adults without previous history of the disorder [57]. These studies may indicate that at least some of the ADHD cases are not related to neurodevelopmental issues. In any case, there are an overwhelming number of studies that suggest a link between the development of the central system and the ADHD. The disturbances related to ADHD are extremely complex, especially given the large number of brain structures involved in the affected processes. Brain imaging techniques have made a critical contribution to deepening our understanding of the neuroanatomical etiology of ADHD. Studies using magnetic resonance have provided us with precise information about the volume of gray matter, density, cortical thickness or integrity of white matter, as well as its connectivity [58–60]. Neuroanatomical development varies throughout childhood until reaching the adult stage, in some cases in a linear fashion, such as the increase in cortical white matter, and in others in an inverted U-shape from the pre-pubertal phase until entering the adult phase, as in the case of cortical gray matter thickness [58]. In addition, this maturation is also carried out unevenly between areas, generally beginning development earlier in the older phylogenetic zones than in the more recent ones, as occurs in the prefrontal cortex. This is also the case in the motor and sensory areas, where development begins earlier than in areas associated with more complex functions, such as those involving cognitive control or attention [58, 59]. These findings are important because an altered maturation process of these latter cortical areas has been identified in patients with ADHD [61], mainly in the frontal cortex [62]. In fact, it has been described that the symptomatology of ADHD in the general population is negatively correlated with total brain size [63], probably due to the decrease in the volume of gray matter in various subcortical structures such as accumbens, amygdala, caudate, hippocampus and putamen; and cortical structures such as the prefrontal cortex and parietal–temporal [63–65]. This decrease is also accompanied by a delay in maturation [66], and is usually more pronounced in childhood, with some persistent reductions in frontal areas in a subgroup of ADHD patients with symptoms lasting into adulthood.

At the functional level, it is observed some correlates that indicate variations in patients with ADHD in relation to patients without a diagnosis of this disorder. For instance, the cortical and subcortical areas described above fluctuate spontaneously when passing from a resting phase to an explicit task phase. The active networks in the resting state reduce their activity when they increase the focused attention processes, with both networks showing a process of negative feedback depending on attentional demands [67–69]. This inverse correlation between the networks of cognitive control and those of rest are diminished or absent in children and adults with ADHD, which is why they show the continuous problems of sustained attention [68, 70, 71]. Furthermore, it is possible, that the connectivity patterns of cortico-limbic, cortico-striatal, and thalamocortical loops are altered in children with ADHD [68, 72]. Specifically, a decrease in the activation of the network connecting the frontal and neostriatal areas next to the thalamus-parietal is observed in ADHD children in goal-directed tasks; although the most common alterations show patterns of hypoactivation of the frontoparietal network, a network related to executive functions [73]. Similarly, the motor inhibition tasks also produce consistent decreases in children diagnosed with ADHD in the associative and sensorimotor network, networks that include the supplementary motor area, anterior cingulate gyrus, and the putamen and caudate nuclei [73, 74].

2.5 Genetic profile in ADHD

The heritability for ADHD has been estimated between 70 to 90% from studies using families and twins with ADHD [75, 76]. By DSM 5, the heritability of ADHD is considerable, being more frequent among first-degree biological relatives of individuals with the disorder. Although ADHD is not associated with specific physical traits, the manual indicates that the presence of minor physical abnormalities such as hypertelorism, bowed palate and low ears, are common among these individuals [1].

Clinical research in ADHD has also identified several genes associated with the disorder which are related to the metabolism, transport and reception of certain neurotransmitters, especially dopamine, noradrenaline and serotonin. Among the genes that have been most frequently correlated with ADHD are the serotonin transport gene 5-HTT and the serotonin receptor gene HTR1B. Regarding dopamine: the DAT1 transporter gene and the DRD2, DRD4 and DRD5 receptor genes; and the gene responsible for the conversion of dopamine into noradrenaline DBH, among others [77–80]. This genetic involvement at the neurotransmitter level would be at the basis of hypofrontality, or reduced activity in the frontal lobes in these patients [81–83]. The frontoparietal network is usually more affected in subjects with an inattentive subtype while in the hyperactive–impulsive type it is usually the frontostriatal network [84]. These dysfunctions have also been found in frontoparietotemporal, frontocerebellar and even frontolimbic circuits [85].

The approaches to the genetics of ADHD have been many and varied. Some studies have found an altered maturation of the cortex, characterized by a delay in cortical maturation in people with ADHD [61, 86]. A study with 366 subjects with a diagnosis of ADHD and a large control group (n = 1047), analyzed the genetics of the disorder by calculating the variation in the copy number of certain genes. The authors found a difference that they called rare in 50 of the 366 subjects with the disorder, 13.66% of the participants with ADHD. In the control group, the abnormality was present in 75 of 1047 cases (7.16%) [87]. It is curious to argue that these differences could be good predictors of the possible genetic origin of the disorder; however, they also found similar results with other diseases, as autism or schizophrenia. And recently, it has been published what is considered to be the largest genetic study of ADHD. Researchers from around the world have participated in the project and it has been proposed as the first gene map around ADHD that identifies variants surpassing genome-wide significance in 12 independent loci. These findings, described by the authors, "are compelling, but only capture a tiny fraction of common variant risk for ADHD" [88]. Furthermore, the contribution of these genes to ADHD heritability is very low [89] and recent studies suggest that we have to look at how the different genes interact each other and with environmental etiological factors [90].

Although technological progress in recent decades has enabled great and important advances in understanding the genetic disposition and physiological and behavioral functioning of many disorders, biological markers for the disorder are still lacking. According to APA "Although specific genes have been correlated with ADHD, these are neither necessary nor sufficient causal factors" [1].

3. Searching a specific phenotype across measurable traits

Above we have discussed about ADHD definition and the difficulties when we try to carry out an accurate diagnosis. In addition, we have indicated that, regardless the diagnosis, the medical care is usually the same. That is, we should not need to differentiate between diagnoses in order to choose a treatment. An alternative to this traditional view of current diagnostic scales could be the objective quantification of specific features that reflect a mental disorder. In this regard, we should give up the idea of how many symptoms are met per patient to be diagnosed of ADHD, and keen on objective scales of how deep is a symptom. In addition, data from genetic studies and brain activity could help us to define the profile of different disorders. This is important because it would allow us to link these measures with quantifiable cognitive/behavioral features in order to develop a possible endophenotype.

One important line of research has identified EEG-based markers as event-related potential and frequency analysis. The use of these markers may improve the diagnosis by offering an alternative to the present symptom-based system. At present, the benefit of using neurofeedback EGG on ADHD is controversial [91, 92]. Although studies on the use of EEG to identify biomarkers related to ADHD is promising, at the moment there are several difficulties. One of the main challenges is defining the ADHD population and the different sub-groups [93]. An alternative to EEG-based markers comes from studies from experimental psychology. For more than a century, the experimental psychology has described the basis of the psychological processes in multiple paradigms. As the ADHD is not a unified disorder, we propose to disentangle some traits related to the ADHD and apply the models from experimental psychology.

4. ADHD focused on impulsivity

Attention is a basic psychological process that facilitates the control of cognitive processes. Traditionally, the distinction made between different dimensions of attention in current models has been associated with different neural networks. Therefore, when we talk about attention we do not talk about a unitary concept [94, 95]. One of the most complete models about attention processes is the one proposed by Posner and Petersen [96]. In its different formulations, it has conceptually modified the basic principles of its original proposal and currently allows to distinguish between several attentional functions. Specifically, it proposes the existence of three networks: the orientation network, the alert network and finally the executive control network. Each one of them would have its own function, supported by an associated brain circuit and mediated by a different neuromodulator. This model has been extended and reformulated in several occasions, highlighting the value of studies that emphasize individual differences between groups of subjects [97].

The executive network has been directly related to goal-directed processes, frontality and action control. Not surprisingly, attention disorders and hyperactivity/impulsivity have gone hand in hand. Thus, when hyperactivity or impulsivity is suspected, its effect on attention is habitually analyzed. However, we do not currently know if the attentional disorders are cause, effect or simply part of shared circuits in ADHD.

The explanatory models range go from those that propose ADHD as the affectation of a single aspect related to the inhibition of response, to models that propose that the disorder is the sum of multiple deficits [98]. Single deficit proposals are related to low capacity in inhibitory control, state regulation and delay avoidance. Specifically, it is related to the lack of capacity to inhibit a response to an attractive and irresistible stimulus associated with immediate reinforcement [2]. In addition, this trait is associated with behavioral impairment of non-verbal working memory, language internalization, and self-regulation on which such inhibition is partially dependent. In other words, ADHD is probably not due to deficits in the processes, but rather to the regulation and control done over those processes.

Impulsive processes have usually been described in at least two different ways. One of them refers to a slow way that involves deliberation and action even considering its negative consequences. The other is the fast way; that is, without thinking of short- or long-term outcomes [99]. This has been translated into two models generally known as cool vs. hot, top-down vs. bottom-up, stopping vs. waiting, action restraint vs. action cancelation or motor vs. choice [100, 101]. Thus, the motor component reflects spontaneity or action without thinking, while unplanned impulsivity reflects a lack of reflection on future consequences. This activity is easily measurable in both human and animal models. In fact, it has been used to analyze patients with ADHD [102]. This view transforms the analysis of impulsive behavior in a quantitative dimension [103], which allows a quantification of the level of impulsivity of individuals, both in human and non-human models, depending on both internal and external variables. This is important because it allows us the study of models of impulsivity from the current theories of learning.

4.1 Impulse control and cognitive correlates in ADHD diagnose

Impulse control is one of the main and consistently affected function in the scientific literature on ADHD [82, 104–107], and it is also one of the difficulties more often reported by parents of boys and girls with ADHD [25]. Accounted as one of the key affectations in ADHD [108, 109], good abilities in impulse control are considered decisive in the future development of individuals [110, 111]. Despite being a common problem among ADHD diagnosed patients, it is more frequently found in people with diagnosed of combined subtype [55].

In addition, these patients show general deficits on working memory [112], and is considered as one of the main alterations and possible axes of the disorder [2, 82].

The central executive appears to be one of the more affected dimensions [113], as well as visuospatial skills [81, 84, 114]. Some authors have found that the greatest deficits in working memory in ADHD were related to tasks involving the central executive [115], while others have proposed that lower performance level in tasks related to executive functions could be explained by deficits in discrimination of interferences in working memory [116]. Interference control is more compromised in subjects with ADHD than in typically developing individuals [117, 118] and visual perception is highly related to higher cognitive processes such as reading comprehension and arithmetic skills [119]. In addition, people with ADHD usually show deficits in tasks that assess visual working memory [120, 121], alterations in visuospatial skills related to working memory [122], and in the ability to process spatial information adequately [123]. However, we do not have standardized tests focused on quantification of the deficit, only a qualitative view of the deficit itself. This might be the reason why it has not found any differences between subtypes of the disorder for this domain yet [124].

Deficits in attention, impulse control, or working memory are just some of the neuropsychological findings in patients with ADHD. Planning and problem solving have also been pointed above as a common deficit in the disorder [82, 125–127], as well as timing skills [128–130], which have also been linked to problems with attention, language, reading and executive functions [131].

Despite the numerous findings identified in the neuropsychology of ADHD, on the one hand, the disturbances expected for the diagnosis not always are found in the assessment process [41]. In addition, they are not only present in this disorder but also in other conditions. Furthermore, the neuropsychological deficits profiles identified are also present in the general population, but in children with ADHD the values are utmost [132].

4.2 Starting the route from animal models

Research in animal models offers an in-depth approach to the possible etiology and development of some diseases, being considered invaluable for the preclinical evaluation of treatments and interventions [133]. In this way, it is generally agreed that those disorders that have previously been studied from the perspective of animal models are currently better understood than others [134]. In this regard, animal models of ADHD, as other brain disorders, need to meet certain characteristics of validity, essential to be considered as an adequate animal model. Similar behavioral characteristics of the disorder are usually known as "face validity". When models show a theoretical consistency with the disorder or disease, we speak of "construct validity". Finally, for being an adequate model, neuroscientific findings, for instance genetic and neurobiology data, should be similar to those displayed in clinical population of the disease in order to ensure "predictive validity" [135, 136].

One of the most analyzed traits studied in animal models has been impulsivity. This is an easy trait to measure at cognitive or behavioral level, besides being closely linked to attention. Recent studies have been able to link different behavioral procedures in order to define possible attentional deficit profile. And these procedures can be used in both, human and non-human animal models, allowing us a quantifiable view of symptoms, making access a deeper view of the disorder.

Autoshaping is currently considered as a valid animal model of impulsivity [137]. This model is based on the study of the motivational aspects of the relationships between the presentation of a conditioned stimulus (CS), the responses to the presence of this stimulus and, finally, the presentation of the unconditioned stimulus (US). The autoshaping, also denominated as sign-tracking, describes the progression of direct movements of orientation-approach to the key or CS that precedes the US [138, 139]. This model allows differentiating how each experimental subject attributes the motivational salience of the signal and the reward, and it is beginning to be used with the aim of assessing individual differences. López et at. [140], studied the behavioral profile in animals classified as sign (ST) and goal (GT) trackers in order to analyze the relationship between impulsivity and attentional processes. Results in prepulse inhibition (PPI), a procedure used to analyze early attentional gating mechanisms, showed a consistent decrease in PPI response in ST animals. That is, animals with a trend to show an impulsive behavior displayed a deficit in a preattentional phase, indicating the more impulsive behavior the higher deficits probability in early phases of attentional process.

Using the same paradigm, Serrano et al. [141] found processing differences of a CS in latent inhibition (LI), other easily quantifiable procedure. LI is a learning process associated to selective attention assessment. This procedure consists in a repeated display of a stimulus without consequences, and after a habituation period, the stimulus is associated to a reward/punishment. The CS-US association tends to be slower in this situation in general population. Yet, animals classified as impulsive (that is, ST) showed a low LI. That is, impulsive animals displayed a slower habituation rate to a neutral stimulus, indicating impulsive animals had paid attention to a higher number of irrelevant stimuli than the rest of population.

The procedures describe above are focused on the named hot model of impulsivity [139]. This kind of impulsivity is usually shown by ST animals, and it is closely related to dopamine neurotransmitter. In fact, nucleus accumbens shows higher levels of dopamine release in the presence of a CS [142]. Besides, D2 dopamine receptors stimulation reduces ST behavior selectively, in a similar way to medial prefrontal cortex lesion [140, 141]. Thus, this model integrates information at different level from this animal model that cover biochemical, anatomical and behavioral level. In this regard, all these data might indicate a higher vulnerability to attentional problems as described in ADHD in impulsive animals.

5. Conclusions

One of the major challenges in the treatment of psychological and psychiatric disorders is to understand the influence of individual differences or traits variability on the potential outcome of treatment. A future goal could be to tailor the treatment to fit the patient profile, rather than assuming a generic approach based on a broad diagnosis. Moreover, many ADHD patients change to more severe clinical diagnosis when they reached adolescence or late adolescence. In this regard the detection of risk factor is essential to focus on detecting what symptom could be a risk factor of possible mental illness in the future. The search of a specific drug for the treatment of different types of ADHD makes increasingly evident the necessity to measure multiple domains of brain and behavior. Here we highlight an alternative to traditional diagnosis scales that would allow a better accurate treatment, regardless of the general symptoms shown.

Acknowledgments

This research was supported by PID2019-110739GB-I00 (Ministerio de Ciencia, Innovación y Universidades, FEDER, UE).

Author details

Annabel Jiménez-Soto, Juan Pedro Vargas, Estrella Díaz and Juan Carlos López*
Animal Behavior and Neuroscience Lab, Universidad de Sevilla, C/Camilo José Cela s/n, Seville, Spain

*Address all correspondence to: jclopez@us.es

References

[1] American Psychiatric Association. Diagnostic and Statistical Manual of Mental Disorders. 5th ed. Washington DC: APA; 2013.

[2] Barkley RA. Behavioral inhibition, sustained attention, and executive functions: Constructing a unifying theory of ADHD. Psychol Bulletin. 1997; 121(1):65-94. DOI: 10.1037/0033-2909.121.1.65

[3] Sonuga-Barke EJS, Taylor E, Sembi S, Smith J. Hyperactivity and delay aversion—I. The effect of delay on choice. J Child Psychol Psychiatry. 1992; 33(2):387-98. DOI: 10.1111/j.1469-7610.1992.tb00874.x

[4] Nielsen M. ADHD and temporality: A desynchronized way of being in the world. Med Anthropol Cross Cult Stud Heal Illn. 2017; 36(3):260-72. DOI: 10.1080/01459740.2016.1274750

[5] Sergeant J. The cognitive-energetic model: An empirical approach to Attention-Deficit Hyperactivity Disorder. Neuroscience and Biobehavioral Reviews. 2000; 24(1):7-12. DOI: 10.1016/S0149-7634(99)00060-3

[6] Barkley RA, Peters H. The earliest reference to ADHD in the medical literature? Melchior Adam Weikard's description in 1775 of "Attention Deficit" (Mangel der Aufmerksamkeit, Attentio Volubilis). J Atten Disord. 2012; 16(8):623-30. DOI: 10.1177/1087054711432309

[7] Lange KW, Reichl S, Lange KM, Tucha L, Tucha O. The history of attention deficit hyperactivity disorder. ADHD. Atten Deficit Hyperact Disord. 2010;2(4):241-55. DOI: 10.1007/s12402-010-0045-8

[8] Thome J, Jacobs KA. Attention deficit hyperactivity disorder (ADHD) in a 19th century children's book. Eur Psychiatry. 2004; 19(5):303-6. DOI: 10.1016/j.eurpsy.2004.05.004

[9] American Psychiatric Association. Diagnostic and Statistical Manual of Mental Disorders. 2nd ed. Washington DC: APA; 1968.

[10] American Psychiatric Association. Diagnostic and Statistical Manual of Mental Disorders. 3rd ed. Washington DC: APA; 1980.

[11] American Psychiatric Association. Diagnostic and Statistical Manual of Mental Disorders. 3rd ed. Rev. Washington DC: APA; 1987.

[12] American Psychiatric Association. Diagnostic and Statistical Manual of Mental Disorders. 4th ed. Washington DC: APA; 1994.

[13] American Psychiatric Association. Diagnostic and Statistical Manual of Mental Disorders. 4th ed. Rev. Washington DC: APA; 2000.

[14] World Health Organization. ICD-10: International Statistical Classification of Diseases and Related Health Problems. 10th Revision. Geneva: World Health Organization; 2004.

[15] World Health Organization. ICD-11 for mortality and morbidity statistics. Available from: https://icd.who.int/browse11/l-m/en [Accessed: 2020-10-09]

[16] American Academy of Pediatrics. Clinical practice guideline: Diagnosis and evaluation of the child with Attention-Deficit/Hyperactivity Disorder. Pediatrics. 2000; 105(5):1158-70. DOI: 10.1542/peds.105.5.1158

[17] American Academy of Child and Adolescent Psychiatry. Practice parameter for the assessment and

treatment of children and adolescents with Attention-Deficit/Hyperactivity Disorder. J Am Acad Child Adolesc Psychiatry. 2007; 46(7):894-921. DOI: 10.1097/chi.0b013e318054e724

[18] Canadian Attention Deficit Hyperactivity Disorder Resource Alliance. CADDRA. Canadian ADHD Practice Guidelines. 3rd ed. Toronto: CADRA; 2011.

[19] Scottish Intercollegiate Guidelines Network (SIGN). Attention deficit and hyperkinetic disorders in children and young people: A national clinical guideline. Edinburgh: SIGN; 2005.

[20] Bruchmüller K, Margraf J, Schneider S. Is ADHD diagnosed in accord with diagnostic criteria? Overdiagnosis and influence of client gender on diagnosis. J Consult Clin Psychol. 2012; 80(1):128-38. DOI: 10.1037/a0026582

[21] Whalen KC. Hiperactividad, problemas de aprendizaje y trastornos por déficit de atención. In: Ollendick T, Hersen S, editors. Psicopatología Infantil. Barcelona: Editorial Martínez Roca; 1986. p. 213-79.

[22] Hartung CM, Lefler EK, Tempel AB, Armendariz ML, Sigel BA, Little CS. Halo effects in ratings of ADHD and ODD: Identification of susceptible symptoms. J Psychopathol Behav Assess. 2010; 32(1):128-37. DOI: 10.1007/s10862-009-9135-3

[23] Fernández-Perrone AL, Fernández-Mayoralas DM, Fernández-Jaén A. Trastorno por déficit de atención/hiperactividad: del tipo inatento al tipo restrictivo. Rev de Neurología. 2013; 56(1):77-84. DOI: 10.33588/rn.56s01.2012651

[24] Canals J, Morales-Hidalgo P, Jané MC, Domènech E. ADHD prevalence in Spanish preschoolers: Comorbidity, socio-demographic factors, and functional consequences. J Atten Disord. 2018; 22(2):143-53. DOI: 10.1177/1087054716638511

[25] McCandless S, O'Laughlin L. The clinical utility of the Behavior Rating Inventory of Executive Function (BRIEF) in the diagnosis of ADHD. J Atten Disord. 2007; 10(4):381-9. DOI: 10.1177/1087054706292115

[26] Applegate B, Lahey BB, Hart EL, Biederman J, Hynd GW, Barkley RA, et al. Validity of the age-of-onset criterion for ADHD: A report from the DSM- IV field trials. J Am Acad Child Adolesc Psychiatry. 1997; 36(9):1211-21. DOI: 10.1097/00004583-199709000-00013

[27] Biederman J, Petty CR, Evans M, Small J, Faraone SV. How persistent is ADHD? A controlled 10-year follow-up study of boys with ADHD. Psychiatry Res. 2010; 177(3):299-304. DOI: 10.1016/j.psychres.2009.12.010

[28] Faraone SV, Biederman J, Mick E. The age-dependent decline of attention deficit hyperactivity disorder: A meta-analysis of follow-up studies. Psychological Medicine. Cambridge University Press. 2006; 36:159-65. DOI: 10.1017/S003329170500471X

[29] Caye A, Rocha TBM, Anselmi L, Murray J, Menezes AMB, Barros FC, et al. Attention-Deficit/Hyperactivity Disorder trajectories from childhood to young adulthood: Evidence from a birth cohort supporting a late-onset syndrome. JAMA Psychiatry. 2016; 73(7):705-12. DOI: 10.1001/jamapsychiatry.2016.0383

[30] Lecendreux M, Silverstein M, Konofal E, Cortese S, Faraone SV. A 9-Year follow-up of Attention-Deficit/Hyperactivity Disorder in a population sample. J Clin Psychiatry. 2019; 80(3). DOI: 10.4088/jcp.18m12642

[31] Capdevila-BrophyC,Artigas-PallarésJ, Ramírez-Mallafré A, López-Rosendo M, Real-Gatius J, Obiols-Llandrich JE. Fenotipo neuropsicológico del trastorno de déficit atencional/hiperactividad: ¿existen diferencias entre los subtipos? Rev Neurol. 2005; 40(S01):S017-23. DOI: 10.33588/rn.40s01.2005074

[32] Nigg JT, Blaskey LG, Huang-Pollock CL, Rappley MD. Neuropsychological Executive Functions and DSM-IV ADHD subtypes. J Am Acad Child Adolesc Psychiatry. 2002;41(1):59-66. DOI: 10.1097/00004583-200201000-00012

[33] Corrigan MW. Debunking ADHD: 10 Reasons to Stop Drugging Kids for Acting Like Kids. New York: Rowman y Littlefield Publishers; 2014.

[34] Ghanizadeh A. Psychiatric comorbidity differences in clinic-referred children and adolescents with ADHD according to the subtypes and gender. J Child Neurol. 2009; 24(6):679-84. DOI: 10.1177/0883073808331086

[35] Brown TE. ADHD Comorbidities: Handbook for ADHD Complications in Children and Adults. Washingtong DC: APA; 2010.

[36] Maedgen JW, Carlson CL. Social functioning and emotional regulation in the Attention Deficit Hyperactivity Disorder subtypes. J Clin Child Adolesc Psychol. 2000; 29(1):30-42. DOI: 10.1207/s15374424jccp2901_4

[37] Michielsen M, Comijs HC, Semeijn EJ, Beekman ATF, Deeg DJH, Kooij JJS. The comorbidity of anxiety and depressive symptoms in older adults with attention-deficit/hyperactivity disorder: A longitudinal study. J Affect Disord. 2013; 148(2-3):220-7. DOI: 10.1016/j.jad.2012.11.063

[38] Septier M, Stordeur C, Zhang J, Delorme R, Cortese S. Association between suicidal spectrum behaviors and Attention-Deficit/Hyperactivity Disorder: A systematic review and meta-analysis. Neurosci and Biobehavioral Reviews. 2019; 103:109-18. DOI: 10.1016/j.neubiorev.2019.05.022

[39] Reale L, Bartoli B, Cartabia M, Zanetti M, Costantino MA, Canevini MP, et al. Comorbidity prevalence and treatment outcome in children and adolescents with ADHD. Eur Child Adolesc Psychiatry. 2017; 26(12):1443-57. DOI: 10.1007/s00787-017-1005-z

[40] Katzman MA, Bilkey TS, Chokka PR, Fallu A, Klassen LJ. Adult ADHD and comorbid disorders: Clinical implications of a dimensional approach. BMC Psychiatry. 2017; 17:302. DOI: 10.1186/s12888-017-1463-3

[41] Jiménez-Soto A. Batería Informatizada para la Evaluación Neuropsicológica de las Afectaciones Relacionadas con el TDAH: BIENART [thesis]. Sevilla: Universidad de Sevilla. 2020.

[42] Lasa-Zulueta A, Jorquera-Cuevas C. Evaluación de la situación asistencial y recomendaciones terapéuticas en el trastorno por déficit de atención e hiperactividad. Informes de Evaluación de Tecnologías Sanitarias: OSTEBA. Vitoria-Gasteiz: Serv. Central de Comunicaciones del Gobierno Vasco; 2010.

[43] García de Vinuesa F, González-Pardo H, Pérez-Álvarez M. Volviendo a la normalidad: La invención del TDAH y del trastorno bipolar infantil. Madrid: Alianza Editorial; 2014.

[44] Batstra L, Nieweg EH, Hadders-Algra M. Exploring five common assumptions on Attention Deficit Hyperactivity Disorder. Acta Paediatrica. International Journal of

Paediatrics. 2014; 103(7): 696-700. DOI: 10.1111/apa.12642

[45] Pérez-Álvarez M. Más Aristóteles y menos Concerta®: Las cuatro causas del TDAH. Ulzama: Ned Ediciones; 2018.

[46] Schwartz A. ADHD nation: Children, doctors, big pharma, and the making of an American epidemic. New York: Simon & Schuster; 2016.

[47] Ainslie G. Specious reward: A behavioral theory of impulsiveness and impulse control. Psychol Bull. 1975; 82(4):463-96.

[48] Eysenck HJ. The nature of impulsivity. In: McCown WG, Johnson JL, Shure MB, editors. The impulsive client: Theory, research, and treatment. Washington DC: American Psychological Association; 1993. p. 57-69. DOI: 10.1037/10500-004

[49] Moeller FG, Barratt ES, Dougherty DM, Schmitz JM, Swann AC. Psychiatric aspects of impulsivity. American Journal of Psychiatry. 2001; 158(11):1783-93. DOI: 10.1176/appi.ajp.158.11.1783

[50] Hofmann W, Friese M, Strack F. Impulse and Self-Control from a Dual-Systems Perspective. Perspect Psychol Sci. 2009; 4(2):162-76. DOI: 10.1111/j.1745-6924.2009.01116.x

[51] Metcalfe J, Mischel W. A hot/cool-system analysis of delay of gratification: Dynamics of willpower. Psychol Rev. 1999; 106(1):3-19. DOI: 10.1037/0033-295X.106.1.3

[52] Allan DM, Lonigan CJ. Examination of the structure and measurement of inattentive, hyperactive, and impulsive behaviors from Preschool to Grade 4. J Abnorm Child Psychol. 2019; 47(6):975-87. DOI: 10.1007/s10802-018-0491-x

[53] Gratch LO. El trastorno por déficit de atención (ADD-ADHD). Clínica, diagnóstico y tratamiento en la infancia, la adolescencia y la adultez. Buenos Aires: Médica Panamericana; 2009.

[54] Rowland AS, Skipper B, Rabiner DL, Umbach DM, Stallone L, Campbell RA, et al. The shifting subtypes of ADHD: Classification depends on how symptom reports are combined. J Abnorm Child Psychol. 2008; 36(5):731-43. DOI: 10.1007/s10802-007-9203-7

[55] Ramos-Galarza C, Pérez-Salas C. Control inhibitorio y monitorización en población infantil con TDAH. Avances en Psicología Latinoam. 2017; 35(1):117-30. DOI: 10.12804/revistas.urosario.edu.co/apl/a.4195

[56] Molina BSG, Hinshaw SP, Swanson JM, Arnold LE, Vitiello B, Jensen PS, et al. The MTA at 8 years: Prospective follow-up of children treated for combined-type ADHD in a multisite study. J Am Acad Child Adolesc Psychiatry. 2009; 48(5):484-500.

[57] Agnew-Blais J, Arseneault L. Late-onset ADHD: Case closed or open question? Am J Psychiatry. 2018; 175(5):481-482. DOI: 10.1176/appi.ajp.2018.17111240

[58] Gogtay N, Giedd JN, Lusk L, Hayashi KM, Greenstein D, Vaituzis AC, et al. Dynamic mapping of human cortical development during childhood through early adulthood. Proc Natl Acad Sci USA. 2004; 101(21):8174-9. DOI: 10.1073/pnas.0402680101

[59] Sowell ER, Peterson BS, Thompson PM, Welcome SE, Henkenius AL, Toga AW. Mapping cortical change across the human life span. Nature Neuroscience. 2003; 6(3):309-15. DOI: 10.1038/nn1008

[60] Sowell ER, Trauner DA, Gamst A, Jernigan TL. Development of cortical and subcortical brain structures in childhood and adolescence: A structural

MRI study. Dev Med Child Neurol. 2007; 44(1):4-16. DOI: 10.1111/j.1469-8749.2002.tb00253.x

[61] Shaw P, Malek M, Watson B, Sharp W, Evans A, Greenstein D. Development of cortical surface area and gyrification in Attention-Deficit/Hyperactivity Disorder. Biol Psychiatry. 2012; 72(3):191-7. DOI: 10.1016/j.biopsych.2012.01.031

[62] Ambrosino S, De Zeeuw P, Wierenga LM, Van Dijk S, Durston S. What can cortical development in Attention-Deficit/Hyperactivity Disorder teach us about the early developmental mechanisms involved? Cereb Cortex. 2017; 27(9):4624-34. DOI: 10.1093/cercor/bhx182

[63] Hoogman M, Rijpkema M, Janss L, Brunner H, Fernandez G, Buitelaar J, et al. Current self-reported symptoms of attention Deficit/Hyperactivity Disorder are associated with total brain volume in healthy adults. PLoS One. 2012; 7(2):e31273. DOI: 10.1371/journal.pone.0031273

[64] Greven CU, Bralten J, Mennes M, O'Dwyer L, Van Hulzen KJE, Rommelse N, et al. Developmentally stable whole-brain volume reductions and developmentally sensitive caudate and putamen volume alterations in those with Attention-Deficit/Hyperactivity Disorder and their unaffected siblings. JAMA Psychiatry. 2015; 72(5):490-9. DOI: 10.1001/jamapsychiatry.2014.3162

[65] Huang-Pollock C, Ratcliff R, McKoon G, Shapiro Z, Weigard A, Galloway-Long H. Using the Diffusion Model to explain cognitive deficits in Attention Deficit Hyperactivity Disorder. J Abnorm Child Psychol. 2017; 45(1):57-68. DOI: 10.1007/s10802-016-0151-y

[66] Hoogman M, Bralten J, Hibar DP, Mennes M, Zwiers MP, Schweren LSJ, et al. Subcortical brain volume differences in participants with Attention Deficit Hyperactivity Disorder in children and adults: a cross-sectional mega-analysis. The Lancet Psychiatry. 2017; 4(4):310-9. DOI: 10.1016/S2215-0366(17)30049-4

[67] Buckner RL, Andrews-Hanna JR, Schacter DL. The brain's default network: Anatomy, function, and relevance to disease. Annals of the New York Academy of Sciences. 2008; 1124:1-38. DOI: 10.1196/annals.1440.011

[68] Posner MI, Rothbart MK, Sheese BE, Voelker P. Developing attention: Behavioral and brain mechanisms. Adv Neuroscience. 2014; 2014(1):1-9. DOI: 10.1155/2014/405094

[69] Raichle ME, Snyder AZ. A default mode of brain function: A brief history of an evolving idea. 2007; 37(4):1083-90. DOI: 10.1016/j.neuroimage.2007.02.041

[70] Castellanos FX, Margulies DS, Kelly C, Uddin LQ, Ghaffari M, Kirsch A, et al. Cingulate-precuneus interactions: A new locus of dysfunction in adult Attention-Deficit/Hyperactivity Disorder. Biol Psychiatry. 2008; 63(3):332-7. DOI: 10.1016/j.biopsych.2007.06.025

[71] Sun L, Cao Q, Long X, Sui M, Cao X, Zhu C, et al. Abnormal functional connectivity between the anterior cingulate and the default mode network in drug-naïve boys with Attention Deficit Hyperactivity Disorder. Psychiatry Res - Neuroimaging. 2012; 201(2):120-7. DOI: 10.1016/j.pscychresns.2011.07.001

[72] Bos DJ, Oranje B, Achterberg M, Vlaskamp C, Ambrosino S, de Reus MA, et al. Structural and functional connectivity in children and adolescents with and without Attention Deficit/Hyperactivity

Disorder. J Child Psychol Psychiatry. 2017; 58(7):810-8. DOI: 10.1111/jcpp.12712

[73] Hart H, Radua J, Nakao T, Mataix-Cols D, Rubia K. Meta-analysis of functional magnetic resonance imaging studies of inhibition and attention in Attention-Deficit/Hyperactivity Disorder: Exploring task-specific, stimulant medication, and age effects. JAMA Psychiatry. 2013; 70(2):185-98. DOI: 10.1001/jamapsychiatry.2013.277

[74] Liou YJ, Wei HT, Chen MH, Hsu JW, Huang KL, Bai YM, et al. Risk of traumatic brain injury among children, adolescents, and young adults with Attention-Deficit Hyperactivity Disorder in Taiwan. J Adolesc Heal. 2018; 63(2):233-8. DOI: 10.1016/j.jadohealth.2018.02.012

[75] Larsson H, Dilshad R, Lichtenstein P, Barker ED. Developmental trajectories of DSM-IV symptoms of Attention-Deficit/Hyperactivity Disorder: Genetic effects, family risk and associated psychopathology. J Child Psychol Psychiatry Allied Discip. 2011; 52(9):954-63. DOI: 10.1111/j.1469-7610.2011.02379.x

[76] Faraone S V, Larsson H. Genetics of Attention Deficit Hyperactivity Disorder. Molecular Psychiatry. 2019; 24:562-75. DOI: 10.1038/s41380-018-0070-0

[77] Barr CL, Wigg KG, Bloom S, Schachar R, Tannock R, Roberts W, et al. Further evidence from haplotype analysis for linkage of the dopamine D4 receptor gene and Attention-Deficit Hyperactivity Disorder. Am J Med Genet - Neuropsychiatry. 2000; 96(3):262-7. DOI: 10.1002/1096-8628(20000612)96:3<262::AID-AJMG5>3.0.CO;2-8

[78] Faraone SV, Khan SA. Candidate gene studies of Attention-Deficit/Hyperactivity Disorder. J Clin Psychiatry. 2006; 67(8):13-20.

[79] Rowe DC, Stever C, Giedinghagen LN, Gard J, Cleveland HH, Terris ST, et al. Dopamine DRD4 receptor polymorphism and Attention Deficit Hyperactivity Disorder. Mol Psychiatry. 1998; 3(5):419-26.

[80] Shook D, Brady C, Lee PS, Kenealy L, Murphy ER, Gaillard WD, et al. Effect of dopamine transporter genotype on caudate volume in childhood ADHD and controls. Am J Med Genet Part B Neuropsy Genet. 2011; 156(1):28-35. DOI: 10.1002/ajmg.b.31132

[81] Brown TE. A new understanding of ADHD in children and adults: executive function impairments. Washington DC: Routledge; 2013.

[82] Willcutt EG, Doyle AE, Nigg JT, Faraone SV, Pennington BF. Validity of the executive function theory of Attention-Deficit/Hyperactivity Disorder: A meta-analytic review. Biological Psychiatry. 2005; 57(11):1336-46. DOI: 10.1016/j.biopsych.2005.02.006

[83] Zang YF, Jin Z, Weng XC, Zhang L, Zeng YW, Yang L, et al. Functional MRI in Attention-Deficit Hyperactivity Disorder: Evidence for hypofrontality. Brain Dev. 2005; 27(8):544-50. DOI: 10.1016/j.braindev.2004.11.009

[84] Diamond A. Attention-deficit disorder (Attention-Deficit/Hyperactivity Disorder without hyperactivity): A neurobiologically and behaviorally distinct disorder from Attention-Deficit/Hyperactivity Disorder (with hyperactivity). Dev Psychopatholy. 2005; 17(3):807-25. DOI: 10.1017/S0954579405050388

[85] Rubia K, Alegría AA, Brinson H. Anomalías cerebrales en el trastorno por déficit de atención/hiperactividad: Una

revisión. Rev Neurol. 2014; 58(1):3-18. DOI: 10.33588/rn.58S01.2013570

[86] Shaw P, Eckstrand K, Sharp W, Blumenthal J, Lerch JP, Greenstein D, et al. Attention-Deficit/Hyperactivity Disorder is characterized by a delay in cortical maturation. Proc Natl Acad Sci U S A. 2007; 104(49):19649-54. DOI: 10.1073/pnas.0707741104

[87] Williams NM, Zaharieva I, Martin A, Langley K, Mantripragada K, Fossdal R, et al. Rare chromosomal deletions and duplications in Attention-Deficit Hyperactivity Disorder: A genome-wide analysis. Lancet. 2010; 376(9750):1401-8. DOI: 10.1016/S0140-6736(10)61109-9

[88] Demontis D, Walters RK, Martin J, Mattheisen M, Als TD, Agerbo E, et al. Discovery of the first genome-wide significant risk loci for Attention Deficit/Hyperactivity Disorder. Nat Genet. 2019; 51(1):63-75. DOI: 10.1038/s41588-018-0269-7

[89] Hohmann S, Adamo N, Lahey BB, Faraone SV, Banaschewski T. Genetics in child and adolescent psychiatry: Methodological advances and conceptual issues. Eur Child Adolesc Psychiatry 2015; 24(6):619-634. DOI: 10.1007/s00787-015-0702-8

[90] Cortese S, Coghill D. Twenty years of research on Attention-Deficit/Hyperactivity Disorder (ADHD): Looking back, looking forward Evidence-Based Mental Health 2018; 21(4):173-176. DOI: 10.1136/ebmental-2018-300050

[91] Van Doren J, Arns M, Heinrich H, Vollebregt MA, Strehl U, Loo K. Sustained effects of neurofeedback in ADHD: A systematic review and meta-analysis. Eur Child Adolesc Psychiatry. 2019; 28(3):293-305. doi:10.1007/s00787-018-1121-4

[92] Schönenberg M, Wiedemann E, Schneidt A, Scheeff J, Logemann A, Keune PM, et al. Neurofeedback, sham neurofeedback, and cognitive-behavioural group therapy in adults with attention-deficit hyperactivity disorder: a triple-blind, randomised, controlled trial. The Lancet Psychiatry. 2017; 4(9):673-84. DOI: 10.1016/S2215-0366(17)30291-2

[93] Miranda P, Cox CD, Alexander M, Danev S, Lakey JRT. In quest of pathognomonic/endophenotypic markers of Attention Deficit Hyperactivity Disorder (ADHD): Potential of EEG-based frequency analysis and ERPs to better detect, prevent and manage ADHD. Med Devices (Auckl). 2020; 13:115-137. DOI: 10.2147/mder.S241205

[94] Castillo Villar MD. La Atención. Madrid: Pirámide; 2009.

[95] De la Fuente-Arnanz J, Pousada M. La Atención. Barcelona: Editorial UOC; 2014.

[96] Posner MI, Petersen SE. The attention system of the human brain. Annu Rev Neurosci. 1990; 13(1):25-42. DOI: 10.1146/annurev.ne.13.030190.000325

[97] Petersen SE, Posner MI. The attention system of the human brain: 20 years after. Annu Rev of Neurosci. 2012; 35:73-89. DOI: 10.1146/annurev-neuro-062111-150525

[98] Artigas-Pallarés J. Modelos cognitivos en el trastorno por déficit de atención/hiperactividad. Rev Neurol. 2009; 49(11):587-93. DOI: 10.33588/rn.4911.2009369

[99] DeYoung CG. Impulsivity as a personality trait. In: Vohs KD, Baumeister RF, editors. Handbook of self-regulation: Research, theory, and applications. New York: Guildford Press; 2011. p. 485-502.

[100] Castellanos FX, Sonuga-Barke EJS, Milham MP, Tannock R. Characterizing

cognition in ADHD: Beyond executive dysfunction. Trends in Cognitive Sciences. 2006; 10(3):117-23. DOI: 10.1016/j.tics.2006.01.011

[101] Lawrence A, Clark L, Labuzetta JN, Sahakian B, Vyakarnum S. The innovative brain. Nature. 2008; 456(7219):168-9. DOI: 10.1038/456168a

[102] Solanto MV, Abikoff H, Sonuga-Barke E, Schachar R, Logan GD, Wigal T, et al. The ecological validity of delay aversion and response inhibition as measures of impulsivity in AD/HD: A supplement to the NIMH multimodal treatment study of AD/HD. J Abnorm Child Psychol. 2001; 29(3):215-28. DOI: 10.1023/A:1010329714819

[103] Bari A, Robbins TW. Animal models of ADHD. Current Topics Behavioral Neuroscience. 2011; 7(1):149-85. DOI: 10.1007/7854_2010_102

[104] Ma I, van Duijvenvoorde A, Scheres A. The interaction between reinforcement and inhibitory control in ADHD: A review and research guidelines. Clinical Psychology Review. 2016; 44:94-111. DOI: 10.1016/j.cpr.2016.01.001

[105] Puiu AA, Wudarczyk O, Goerlich KS, Votinov M, Herpertz-Dahlmann B, Turetsky B, et al. Impulsive aggression and response inhibition in attention-deficit/hyperactivity disorder and disruptive behavioral disorders: Findings from a systematic review. Neurosci and Biobehavioral Reviews. 2018; 90: 231-46. DOI: 10.1016/j.neubiorev.2018.04.016

[106] Skogli EW, Egeland J, Andersen PN, Hovik KT, Øie M. Few differences in hot and cold executive functions in children and adolescents with combined and inattentive subtypes of ADHD. Child Neuropsychology. 2014; 20(2):162-81. DOI: 10.1080/09297049.2012.753998

[107] Van Dessel J, Morsink S, Van der Oord S, Lemiere J, Moerkerke M, Grandelis M, et al. Waiting impulsivity: a distinctive feature of ADHD neuropsychology? Child Neuropsychol. 2019; 25(1):122-9. DOI: 10.1080/09297049.2018.1441819

[108] Janssen TWP, Heslenfeld DJ, van Mourik R, Logan GD, Oosterlaan J. Neural correlates of response inhibition in children with Attention-Deficit/Hyperactivity Disorder: A controlled version of the stop-signal task. Psychiatry Res – Neuroimaging. 2015; 233(2):278-84. DOI: 10.1016/j.pscychresns.2015.07.007

[109] Slaats-Willemse D, Swaab-Barneveld H, De Sonneville L, Van Der Meulen E, Buitelaar J. Deficient response inhibition as a cognitive endophenotype of ADHD. J Am Acad Child Adolesc Psychiatry. 2003; 42(10):1242-8. DOI: 10.1097/00004583-200310000-00016

[110] Blair C, Raver CC, Finegood ED. Self-regulation and developmental psychopathology: Experiential canalization of brain and behavior. In: Cicchetti D, editor. Developmental Psychopathology. New Jersey: John Wiley & Sons; 2016. DOI: 10.1002/9781119125556.devpsy213

[111] Ursache A, Blair C, Raver CC. The promotion of self-regulation as a means of enhancing school readiness and early achievement in children at risk for school failure. Child Development Perspectives. 2012; 6(2):122-8. DOI: 10.1111/j.1750-8606.2011.00209.x

[112] Wells EL, Kofler MJ, Soto EF, Schaefer HS, Sarver DE. Assessing working memory in children with ADHD: Minor administration and scoring changes may improve digit span backward's construct validity. Res Dev

Disabil. 2018; 72:166-78. DOI: 10.1016/j.ridd.2017.10.024

[113] Martinussen R, Hayden J, Hogg-Johnson S, Tannock R. A meta-analysis of working memory impairments in children with Attention-Deficit/Hyperactivity Disorder. J Am Acad Child Adolesc Psychiatry. 2005; 44(4):377-84. DOI: 10.1097/01.chi.0000153228.72591.73

[114] Flores JC. Características de comorbilidad en los diferentes subtipos de Trastorno por Déficit de Atención con Hiperactividad. Psicothema. 2009; 21(4), 592-597.

[115] Rapport MD, Alderson RM, Kofler MJ, Sarver DE, Bolden J, Sims V. Working memory deficits in boys with Attention-Deficit/Hyperactivity Disorder (ADHD): The contribution of central executive and subsystem processes. J Abnorm Child Psychol. 2008; 36:825-37. DOI: 10.1007/s10802-008-9215-y

[116] Riccio CA, Homack S, Jarratt KP, Wolfe ME. Differences in academic and executive function domains among children with ADHD Predominantly Inattentive and Combined Types. Arch Clin Neuropsycholy. 2006; 21(7):657-67. DOI: 10.1016/j.acn.2006.05.010

[117] Lansbergen MM, Kenemans JL, Van Engeland H. Stroop interference and Attention-Deficit/Hyperactivity Disorder: A review and meta-analysis. Neuropsychology. 2007; 21(2):251-62. DOI: 10.1037/0894-4105.21.2.251

[118] Sebastian A, Gerdes B, Feige B, Klöppel S, Lange T, Philipsen A, et al. Neural correlates of interference inhibition, action withholding and action cancelation in adult ADHD. Psychiatry Res – Neuroimaging. 2012; 202(2):132-41. DOI: 10.1016/j.pscychresns.2012.02.010

[119] Cui J, Zhang Y, Wan S, Chen C, Zeng J, Zhou X. Visual form perception is fundamental for both reading comprehension and arithmetic computation. Cognition. 2019; 189:141-54. DOI: 10.1016/j.cognition.2019.03.014

[120] Ackermann S, Halfon O, Fornari E, Urben S, Bader M. Cognitive Working Memory Training (CWMT) in adolescents suffering from Attention-Deficit/Hyperactivity Disorder (ADHD): A controlled trial taking into account concomitant medication effects. Psychiatry Res. 2018; 269:79-85. DOI: 10.1016/j.psychres.2018.07.036

[121] Matsuura N, Ishitobi M, Arai S, Kawamura K, Asano M, Inohara K, et al. Distinguishing between Autism Spectrum Disorder and Attention Deficit Hyperactivity Disorder by using behavioral checklists, cognitive assessments, and neuropsychological test battery. Asian J Psychiatry. 2014; 12(1):50-7. DOI: 10.1016/j.ajp.2014.06.011

[122] Alderson MR, Kasper LJ, Hudec KL, Patros CHG. Attention-Deficit/Hyperactivity Disorder (ADHD) and working memory in adults: A meta-analytic review. Neuropsychology. 2013; 27(3):287-302. DOI: 10.1037/a0032371

[123] Tamm L, Juranek J. Fluid reasoning deficits in children with ADHD: Evidence from fMRI. Brain Res. 2012; 1465:48-56. DOI: 10.1016/j.brainres.2012.05.021

[124] Gallego-Martínez A, Fenollar-Cortés J, García-Sevilla J. Implicación de la memoria visoespacial y fonológica en la heterogeneidad clínica del Trastorno por Déficit de Atención con Hiperactividad (TDAH). Anales de Psicol. 2018; 34(1):16-22. DOI: 10.6018/analesps.34.1.289671

[125] Aguiar A, Eubig PA, Schantz SL. Attention Deficit/Hyperactivity Disorder: A focused overview for

children's environmental health researchers. Environmental Health Perspectives. 2010; 118(12):1646-53. DOI: 10.1289/ehp.1002326

[126] Rubiales J. Executive functioning in children with Attention Deficit Hyperactivity Disorder. Rev Iberoam Diagnóstico y Evaluación. 2014;2(38):31-54.

[127] Barkley RA. Attention-Deficit Hyperactivity Disorder: A Handbook for Diagnosis and Treatment. 4th ed. New York: Guilford Publications; 2018.

[128] Falter CM, Noreika V. Time processing in developmental disorders: A comparative view. In: Arstila V, Lloyd D, editors. Subjective time: The philosophy, psychology, and neuroscience of temporality. Cambridge: MIT Press; 2014. p. 557-97.

[129] Toplak ME, Dockstader C, Tannock R. Temporal information processing in ADHD: Findings to date and new methods. J Neurosci Methods. 2006; 151(1):15-29. DOI: 10.1016/j.jneumeth.2005.09.018

[130] Dahan A, Ryder CH, Reiner M. Components of motor deficiencies in ADHD and possible interventions. Neuroscience. 2018; 378:34-53. DOI: 10.1016/j.neuroscience.2016.05.040

[131] Noreika V, Falter CM, Rubia K. Timing deficits in Attention-Deficit/Hyperactivity Disorder (ADHD): Evidence from neurocognitive and neuroimaging studies. Neuropsychologia. 2013; 51(2):235-66. DOI: 10.1016/j.neuropsychologia.2012.09.036

[132] Drechsler R, Brem S, Brandeis D, Grünblatt E, Berger G, Walitza S. ADHD: Current concepts and treatments in children and adolescents. Neuropediatrics. 2020; 51(5):315-35. DOI: 10.1055/s-0040-1701658

[133] Sharma N, Jamwal S, Bansal PK. Animal Models of Attention-Deficit Hyperkinetic Disorder (ADHD). In: Bansal PK, Deshmusk R, editors. Animal Models of Neurological Disorders: Principle and Working Procedure for Animal Models of Neurological Disorders. New York: Springer; 2017. p. 217-32.

[134] Russell VA, Sagvolden T, Johansen EB. Animal models of Attention-Deficit Hyperactivity Disorder. Behavioral and Brain Functions. 2005; 1(9):1-17. DOI: 10.1186/1744-9081-1-9

[135] Escorihuela RM, Fernández-Teruel A. Modelos animales en psicopatología y psicofarmacología: del análisis experimental de la conducta a la neurogenética. Psicología Conductual. 1998; 6(1):165-91.

[136] Sagvolden T, Russell VA, Aase H, Johansen EB, Farshbaf M. Rodent models of Attention-Deficit/Hyperactivity Disorder. Biol Psychiatry. 2005; 57(11):1239-47. DOI: 10.1016/j.biopsych.2005.02.002

[137] Vargas JP, Díaz E, Portavella M, López JC. Animal models of maladaptive traits: Disorders in sensorimotor gating and attentional quantifiable responses as possible endophenotypes. Front Psychol. 2016; 7(206):1-9. DOI: 10.3389/fpsyg.2016.00206

[138] Flagel SB, Watson SJ, Robinson TE, Akil H. Individual differences in the propensity to approach signals vs goals promote different adaptations in the dopamine system of rats. Psychopharmacology. 2007; 191(3):599-607. DOI: 10.1007/s00213-006-0535-8

[139] Robinson TE, Flagel SB. Dissociating the predictive and incentive motivational properties of reward-related cues through the study of individual differences. Biol Psychiatry. 2009; 65(10):869-73.

[140] Lopez JC, Karlsson RM, O'Donnell P. Dopamine D2 modulation of sign and goal tracking in rats. Neuropsychopharmacology. 2015; 40(9):2096-102. DOI: 10.1038/npp.2015.68

[141] Serrano-Barroso A, Vargas JP, Diaz E, O'Donnell P, López JC. Sign and goal tracker rats process differently the incentive salience of a conditioned stimulus. PLoS One. 2019; 14(9):1-16. DOI: 10.1371/journal.pone.0223109

[142] Flagel SB, Clark JJ, Robinson TE, Mayo L, Czuj A, Willuhn I, et al. A selective role for dopamine in stimulus-reward learning. Nature. 2011; 469(7328):53-9. DOI: 10.1038/nature09588

Chapter 3

Role of Copy Number Variations in ADHD

Danijela Krgović

Abstract

Copy number variations (CNV) have an important role in etiology of neurodevelopmental disorders (NDD). Among them, individuals with attention-deficit and hyperactivity disorders (ADHD) have 1.33 times higher overall rate of CNVs larger than 100 kb compared to healthy controls. These CNVs are often shared with other NDDs and neuropsychiatric disorders such as schizophrenia (SCZ) and autism spectrum disorder (ASD), although duplications of 15q13.3 and 16p13.11 have been found enriched in ADHD cohorts. CNVs provide new opportunities for studying and management of psychiatric disorders including ADHD. Therefore this chapter provides a brief overview of the literature on this topic and presents the benefits of CNV genetic diagnostics in ADHD patients.

Keywords: attention-deficit and hyperactivity disorders (ADHD), neuropsychiatric disorders, neurodevelopmental disorders (NDDs), copy number variations (CNV), chromosomal microarrays (CMA), whole genome sequencing (WGS)

1. Introduction

Attention-deficit and hyperactivity disorders (ADHD) is a childhood-onset neuropsychiatric disorder affecting 5–6% of children [1]. The follow-up studies of children with ADHD showed that symptoms are evident even in adulthood in approximately two-third of patients [2] and that disorder is present in 2.5% of adults [1, 3]. The twin studies suggest a high heritability of ADHD, estimated to be at approximately 70% [4]. This is comparable to the heredity of other neuropsychiatric disorders, such as autism spectrum disorder (ASD) and schizophrenia (SCZ) [5]. Genetic studies shown a complex genetic etiology comprising both common variants such are single nucleotide polymorphisms (SNPs) [6], as well as rare variants causing a loss-of-function in single gene in form of single nucleotide variants (SNVs) [7], and deletions or duplications of multiple genes in form of copy number variations (CNVs) [8–10]. A SNP-based genome wide heritability studies can explain the genetic origin of the ADHD in approximately 22% cases, which still does not explain the large proportion of heredity set out in twin studies [6]. To some extent the difference can be explained by rare variants in form of SNVs and CNVs [11].

In 2010, a chromosomal microarrays (CMA) which are used for detection of genomic CNVs, became first-tier clinical diagnostic test for individuals with developmental delay and/or intellectual disability (DD/ID), ASD, and/or multiple congenital anomalies. Namely, a review of 33 studies including 21,698 patients tested by CMA showed that a pathogenic CNV could be determined in an average of 12.2% patients across all studies [12]. Since then, rare CNVs have been described across different neurodevelopmental disorders (NDDs) [13]. In individuals with ADHD a 1.33 times higher overall rate of CNVs larger than 100 kb compared to the healthy controls was observed [14].

Therefore, an important role of CNVs in etiology of ADHD is further discussed in this chapter.

2. What are CNVs?

CNVs are genomic structural variations causing the deletion or duplication of coding and non-coding segments of DNA. They vary in size, spanning from single gene to encompassing multiple genes. They can be common or rare events in genome acting as a disease cause.

CNVs occur in genome due to the segmental duplications present in certain regions in human genome. These repetitive sequences represent CNV "hotspots" as they make these regions prone to mutational mechanism called non-allelic homologs recombination. The process occurs during sperm or egg formation, therefore CNV prevalence remains relatively constant regardless of the severity of genomic disorder [15].

The CMA technology was designed to detect deletions and duplications across human genome randomly, without the need of specific suspected diagnosis of genomic disorder made by clinician. The technology enables us to identify the recurrent as well as novel disease associated CNVs [15]. Rare CNVs have been described as microdeletions or microduplications involved in many NDDs [12, 16–20].

Rare CNVs are considered to be present in less than <0.1% of general population. Disease associated CNVs are rare but collectively explain approximately 20% of DD/ID, 10% of ASD, and 5% of SCZ cases. However for other neuropsychiatric conditions the role of rare CNVs in disease pathophysiology is less clear, therefore diagnostics yield for CMA remains to be determined [17].

An important role in prevalence of rare CNV has its relative overall penetrance. CNVs with high overall penetrance are expected to be absent from general population whereas low penetrance CNVs have higher chance to be found in general population, where CNV carriers may have mild clinical manifestation [21, 22].

Different NDDs also share same CNVs effecting the same genes [4, 17] indicating on their clinical pleiotropy [13].

3. Role of CNVs in ADHD

ADHD has a complex genetic architecture. The larger sample size and advances in technology enabled to study an effect of different classes of genetic variations in disease development. This revealed that ADHD is polygenic disorder like other neuropsychiatric disorders and its genetic architecture involves both the thousands of common variants with individually small effect size (SNPs), as well as rare variants causing a loss-of-function in single gene (SNVs) or small or larger genome deletions or duplications (CNVs) [23]. From all the genetic variants that contribute to etiology of ADHD, CNVs probably have the most evident clinical evidence, since they are enriched in several neuropsychiatric disorders [15].

ADHD is often associated with syndromic disorders [5]. For example, ADHD symptoms are present in more than 60% of patients with Williams-Beuren syndrome caused by microdeletion of chromosome region 7q11.23 [24] and approximately 40% patients with 22q11 deletion syndrome, also known as DiGeorge syndrome [25].

A parent-offspring trio studies showed a higher rate of de novo CNVs in children with NDDs. The highest is observed in 10% of children with ID/DD [26]. For ASD patients a 3- to 5-fold higher rate is observed than in control [27]. Similar rate was observed in SCZ-trio studies [28]. Only recently, studies of ADHD patients have reached the number of patients, which would unable similar studies to be performed as in ASD and SCZ patients [5]. Most recent trio-based study of ADHD patients have shown that overall mutation rate of de novo CNVs was 4.6% and similar to the rate observed in children with ADS, but slightly higher than in SCZ study [29]. Their rate was also higher than from previously trio-based ADHD study, which was 1.7% [30]. From the 14 de novo CNVs found in 13 ADHD probands, four CNVs: duplications of 15q13.1, 16p13.11 and 22q11.21 and deletion of 16p12.1, have been previously implicated in neuropsychiatric disorders or NDDs, once again highlighting their clinical pleiotropy [29].

In the study of Gudmundsson et al., a presence of 19 rare neuropsychiatric CNVs, that confer risk of ASD and SCZ, have been tested in 8883 ADHD probands. Presence was confirmed in 2.15% of individuals, compared to the 0.86% of controls. Only one CNV carrier had comorbid diagnosis of ADHD and ASD, and none for SCZ. Eight of the tested CNVs were significantly associated with ADHD risk: deletion of 2p16.3 (*NRXN1*), 15q11.2, 15q13.3, and 22q11.21 and duplications of 1q21.1 distal, 16p11.2 proximal, 16p13.11, and 22q11.21 [10]. Among them, deletion of DiGeorge region (22q11 deletion) was established to have highest risk of ADHD, since in addition to high frequency of SCZ in DiGeorge patients, ADHD has been observed in 37% of the children [31]. A high significance to ADHD was also confirmed for 15q13.3 deletion. Deletions of this region is associated with various NDDs [32] with the higher rate of neuropsychiatric disorders, along with 6.5% of ADHD [3, 33].

3.1 Does ADHD-specific CNVs exist?

There is still no ADHD-specific CNV identified. Although, there are still some incocistency about frequency of rare CNVs in ADHD patients [30, 34–38], studies of CNVs in ADHD patients show a higher burden of this structural variants compared to the control [8, 9, 30, 39, 40].

The CNVs found in patients with ADHD often coincide with ASD and SCZ chromosomal loci [41–43], which is also evident in clinical comorbidity of ADHD with this two disorders [44]. Stronger comorbidity is set for ASD [45] by common CNV-affected genes [8, 9, 30] and biological pathways [46]. Overlap of the disease-associated genes between ASD and ADHD was also observed in SNVs studies [7].

A large genome-wide CNV analysis was performed recently in 2691 patients diagnosed with different NDDs, in order to determine the pleiotropy of CNVs. For example, genes like *NRXN1*, *EXOC3*, and *PCMTD2* were found in ASD, ADHD and SCZ or ASD, ADHD and obsessive compulsive disorder (OCD) or ASD, OCD and SCH patients respectively. Recurrent and non-recurrent CNV regions were also identified to be involved in multiple NDDs, as 16p13.11 and 15q11-q13 duplications in SCZ, OCD, ASD and ADHD. The study also showed that clinically relevant CNV was detected in 9.4% (N 40/427) ADHD patients, similar to the percentage in ASD (11.4%) and SCZ (10.8%) patients [13]. Studies like this show an importance of CNVs in genetics of NDDs and complex genetic architecture of this disorders.

Interestingly, not much has been done in studying the CNVs implicated in ID/DD, since ADHD patients who have comorbid ID/DD are usually exclude from such studies [23].

A recent study of CNV involved genes obtained from 11 published studies was performed with aim to define ADHD-associated candidate genes. Among 2241 localized genes from 1532 CNVs, 26 genes were established to have highest credibility as ADHD candidate genes. This genes also share common biological topic such as transcription, mitochondrial biology, mRNA metabolism, and cytoskeleton [47].

3.2 Ambiguity of the rare CNVs

By researching of the genome and CNV mapping, it was estimated that sequence included in CNVs contribute to the 4.8–9.5% of the genome. Additionally, it was postulated that about 100 genes can be deleted by CNVs and have no apparent phenotype [19]. Furthermore, an average mutation rate in individuals in the general population should be take into account, consequently rare variants could be false positive [48].

Therefore, the meaning of a rare unknown CNV identified in ADHD patient should be carefully interpreted.

4. The importance of CNV in diagnostics of ADHD

Reaching the genetic diagnosis in ADHD patient can have many advantages for the patient as well as clinician. Molecular diagnosis can benefit in patients' care in management and treatment (e.g. preference or avoidance of particular medications) as well as prognosis [15].

Genetic counseling is also important. The family based and twin studies of ADHD patients revealed a strong familial and genetic overlap of ADHD with ASD and ID. The individuals with monozygotic twin with ASD have an increased risk for ADHD compared to the risk observed in dizygotic twin studies. The association is higher for higher-functioning than lower-functioning ASD [23]. Siblings of ADHD probands have ninefold higher risk to ADHD compared to the siblings in controls [49]. ADHD is also strongly associated with lower IQ and ID indicating that they share heritability [23]. Additionally, family members of ADHD individuals are at elevated risk for neurodevelopmental and neuropsychiatric disorders. Knowing the genetic cause may have an impact on their management and treatment [23].

CNVs will lead to understanding how genes affect biological pathways involved in ADHD. For example, CNVs in glutameric genes were liked to cognitive and clinical impairments of ADHD [4]. In study of Thapar et al. found CNVs in ADHD patients were enriched in genes for which it was previously known to be involved in SCZ, Fragile X ID, and partly with autism [50]. More recently 26 ADHD-associated candidate genes were identified that share common biological topic such as transcription, mitochondrial biology, mRNA metabolism, and cytoskeleton [47].

Other features can be explain by CNVs. The duplications of *CHRNA7* gene were observed in higher rate in ADHD patients [9]. This gene encodes alpha-7 nicotinic acetylcholine receptor. A higher rate of smokers have been observed in ADHD patients [51]. Namely, nicotine administration reduce hyperactivity and impulsivity [52] since nicotine modulates dopaminergic neurons by interacting with nicotinic acetylcholine receptors [53].

Moreover, knowledge of the cause of the disease assist in better understanding and felicitate the acceptance of the condition, improves genetic counseling and also refine possible future new treatments [15].

Although there are still no clear guidelines when to perform genetic testing for rare variants in ADHD patients, testing for CNVs is recommended in individuals with comorbid mild ID or ASD [23].

5. Future prospects

Technologies such as whole genome sequencing (WGS) that enable us to detect SNVs as well as structural variants in the genome in a single experiment, will facilitate the detection of even smaller CNVs, which we could not detect with CMA due to technology limitations.

Pathogenicity of rare large CNVs in NDDs and neuropsychiatric disorders is mostly defined, whereas a significance of a small nonrecurrent CNVs (<500 kb) is still ambiguous. In the study of 4417 patients referred to CMA testing 383 (8.67%) patient had at least one small, nonrecurrent CNV. Of these, 142 (3.21%) patients were carriers of pathogenic or likely pathogenic CNV, from which in 80 patients a single gene or exonic deletion of the gene was found [54].

A CNV study in adult ADHD patients did not found enrichment for large CNVs, however they did found significant increase of small CNVs [14]. Therefore, the relevance of new technologies in studying of genomic disorders will facilitate new genotype–phenotype correlation [15].

6. Conclusions

CNVs provide new opportunities for studying and management of psychiatric disorders including ADHD.

Detection of small CNVs of few kilo base in size is still difficult due to method limitations, although WGS of the ADHD patients promises their discovery. On the other hand, for the detection of large rare CNVs that occurs with frequency less than 1%, large sample size are needed [5].

Furthermore, parent-offspring trio studies of de novo CNVs and SNVs will contribute in disease etiology, since de novo aberrations in genome are more likely deleterious [28]. Identification of disease-associated genes and knowledge of their molecular functions will lead to better understanding of their disease pathology and hopefully enable better diagnostic and treatment [47].

Genetic counseling for polygenic disorders with complex genetic architecture as is ADHD is challenging, due to variable phenotypic outcomes and incomplete penetrance encountered in majority of genetic disorders. Therefore understanding the molecular etiology for clinicians is useful in patient management, in terms of improving risk predictions, screening for extra-psychiatric features, treatment, etc. [15]. New discoveries are also a starting point for identifying and assessing novel treatments in ADHD patients [23].

Though psychiatric genetics is unlikely to change the treatment of patients, it will eventually contribute to more personalized medicine [5]. Therefore the role of CNVs in clinical practice for ADHD patients remains to be seen.

Acknowledgements

My work was supported by the research program P4-0220 Comparative genomics and genomic biodiversity and research project Z3-9294 (B). Advanced genomic analyses of Slovenian children with Autistic Spectrum Disorders from the Slovenian Research Agency (ARRS).

Conflict of interest

No conflict of interest.

Author details

Danijela Krgović[1,2]

1 Division of Gynecology and Perinatology, Medical Genetics Laboratory, University Medical Centre Maribor, Maribor, Slovenia

2 Department of Molecular Biology, Faculty of Medicine, University of Maribor, Maribor, Slovenia

*Address all correspondence to: danijela.krgovic@ukc-mb.si; danijela.krgovic1@um.si

References

[1] Faraone SV, Asherson P, Banaschewski T, Biederman J, Buitelaar JK, Ramos-Quiroga JA, et al. Attention-deficit/hyperactivity disorder. Nature Reviews. Disease Primers. 2015;**1**:15020. DOI: 10.1038/nrdp.2015.20

[2] Franke B, Michelini G, Asherson P, Banaschewski T, Bilbow A, Buitelaar JK, et al. Live fast, die young? A review on the developmental trajectories of ADHD across the lifespan. European Neuropsychopharmacology. 2018;**28**(10):1059-1088. DOI: 10.1016/j.euroneuro.2018.08.001

[3] Franke B, Faraone SV, Asherson P, Buitelaar J, Bau CH, Ramos-Quiroga JA, et al. International multicentre persistent ADHD CollaboraTion: The genetics of attention deficit/hyperactivity disorder in adults, a review. Molecular Psychiatry. 2012;**17**(10):960-987. DOI: 10.1038/mp.2011.138

[4] Faraone SV, Larsson H. Genetics of attention deficit hyperactivity disorder. Molecular Psychiatry. 2019;**24**(4):562-575. DOI: 10.1038/s41380-018-0070-0

[5] Grimm O, Kranz TM, Reif A. Genetics of ADHD: What should the clinician know? Current Psychiatry Reports. 2020 Feb 27;**22**(4):18. DOI: 10.1007/s11920-020-1141-x

[6] Demontis D, Walters RK, Martin J, Mattheisen M, Als TD, Agerbo E, Baldursson G, Belliveau R, Bybjerg-Grauholm J, Bækvad-Hansen M, Cerrato F, Chambert K, Churchhouse C, Dumont A, Eriksson N, Gandal M, Goldstein JI, Grasby KL, Grove J, Gudmundsson OO, Hansen CS, Hauberg ME, Hollegaard MV, Howrigan DP, Huang H, Maller JB, Martin AR, Martin NG, Moran J, Pallesen J, Palmer DS, Pedersen CB, Pedersen MG, Poterba T, Poulsen JB, Ripke S, Robinson EB, Satterstrom FK, Stefansson H, Stevens C, Turley P, Walters GB, Won H, Wright MJ; ADHD Working Group of the Psychiatric Genomics Consortium (PGC); Early Lifecourse & Genetic Epidemiology (EAGLE) Consortium; 23andMe Research Team, Andreassen OA, Asherson P, Burton CL, Boomsma DI, Cormand B, Dalsgaard S, Franke B, Gelernter J, Geschwind D, Hakonarson H, Haavik J, Kranzler HR, Kuntsi J, Langley K, Lesch KP, Middeldorp C, Reif A, Rohde LA, Roussos P, Schachar R, Sklar P, Sonuga-Barke EJS, Sullivan PF, Thapar A, Tung JY, Waldman ID, Medland SE, Stefansson K, Nordentoft M, Hougaard DM, Werge T, Mors O, Mortensen PB, Daly MJ, Faraone SV, Børglum AD, Neale BM: Discovery of the first genome-wide significant risk loci for attention deficit/hyperactivity disorder. Nature Genetics 2019;51(1):63-75. doi: 10.1038/s41588-018-0269-7

[7] Satterstrom FK, Walters RK, Singh T, Wigdor EM, Lescai F, Demontis D, Kosmicki JA, Grove J, Stevens C, Bybjerg-Grauholm J, Bækvad-Hansen M, Palmer DS, Maller JB; iPSYCH-Broad Consortium, Nordentoft M, Mors O, Robinson EB, Hougaard DM, Werge TM, Bo Mortensen P, Neale BM, Børglum AD, Daly MJ: Autism spectrum disorder and attention deficit hyperactivity disorder have a similar burden of rare protein-truncating variants. Nature Neuroscience 2019;22(12):1961-1965. doi: 10.1038/s41593-019-0527-8

[8] Williams NM, Zaharieva I, Martin A, Langley K, Mantripragada K, Fossdal R, et al. Rare chromosomal deletions and duplications in attention-deficit hyperactivity disorder: A genome-wide analysis. Lancet. 2010;**376**(9750):1401-1408. DOI: 10.1016/S0140-6736(10)61109-9

[9] Williams NM, Franke B, Mick E, Anney RJ, Freitag CM, Gill M, et al. Genome-wide analysis of copy number variants in attention deficit hyperactivity disorder: The role of rare variants and duplications at 15q13.3. The American Journal of Psychiatry. 2012;**169**(2):195-204. DOI: 10.1176/appi.ajp.2011.11060822

[10] Gudmundsson OO, Walters GB, Ingason A, Johansson S, Zayats T, Athanasiu L, et al. Attention-deficit hyperactivity disorder shares copy number variant risk with schizophrenia and autism spectrum disorder. Translational Psychiatry. 2019;**9**(1):258. DOI: 10.1038/s41398-019-0599-y

[11] Demontis D, Lescai F, Børglum A, Glerup S, Østergaard SD, Mors O, et al. Whole-exome sequencing reveals increased burden of rare functional and disruptive variants in candidate risk genes in individuals with persistent attention-deficit/hyperactivity disorder. Journal of the American Academy of Child and Adolescent Psychiatry. 2016;**55**(6):521-523. DOI: 10.1016/j.jaac.2016.03.009

[12] Miller DT, Adam MP, Aradhya S, Biesecker LG, Brothman AR, Carter NP, et al. Consensus statement: Chromosomal microarray is a first-tier clinical diagnostic test for individuals with developmental disabilities or congenital anomalies. American Journal of Human Genetics. 2010;**86**(5):749-764. DOI: 10.1016/j.ajhg.2010.04.006

[13] Zarrei M, Burton CL, Engchuan W, Young EJ, Higginbotham EJ, MacDonald JR, et al. A large data resource of genomic copy number variation across neurodevelopmental disorders. NPJ Genomic Medicine. 2019;**4**:26. DOI: 10.1038/s41525-019-0098-3

[14] Ramos-Quiroga JA, Sánchez-Mora C, Casas M, Garcia-Martínez I, Bosch R, Nogueira M, et al. Genome-wide copy number variation analysis in adult attention-deficit and hyperactivity disorder. Journal of Psychiatric Research. 2014;**49**:60-67. DOI: 10.1016/j.jpsychires.2013.10.022

[15] Lowther C, Costain G, Baribeau DA, Bassett AS. Genomic disorders in psychiatry-what does the clinician need to know? Current Psychiatry Reports. 2017;**19**(11):82. DOI: 10.1007/s11920-017-0831-5

[16] Cook EH Jr, Scherer SW. Copy-number variations associated with neuropsychiatric conditions. Nature. 2008 Oct 16;**455**(7215):919-923. DOI: 10.1038/nature07458

[17] Lee C, Scherer SW. The clinical context of copy number variation in the human genome. Expert Reviews in Molecular Medicine. 2010;**12**:e8. DOI: 10.1017/S1462399410001390

[18] Scherer SW, Dawson G. Risk factors for autism: Translating genomic discoveries into diagnostics. Human Genetics. 2011;**130**(1):123-148. DOI: 10.1007/s00439-011-1037-2

[19] Zarrei M, MacDonald JR, Merico D, Scherer SW. A copy number variation map of the human genome. Nature Reviews. Genetics. 2015;**16**(3):172-183. DOI: 10.1038/nrg3871

[20] Smoller JW, Andreassen OA, Edenberg HJ, Faraone SV, Glatt SJ, Kendler KS. Psychiatric genetics and the structure of psychopathology. Molecular Psychiatry. 2019;**24**(3):409-420. DOI: 10.1038/s41380-017-0010-4

[21] Männik K, Mägi R, Macé A, Cole B, Guyatt AL, Shihab HA, et al. Copy number variations and cognitive phenotypes in unselected populations. Journal of the American Medical Association. 2015;**313**(20):2044-2054. DOI: 10.1001/jama.2015.4845

[22] Stefansson H, Meyer-Lindenberg A, Steinberg S, Magnusdottir B, Morgen K, Arnarsdottir S, et al. CNVs conferring risk of autism or schizophrenia affect cognition in controls. Nature. 2014;**505**(7483):361-366. DOI: 10.1038/nature12818

[23] Thapar A. Discoveries on the genetics of ADHD in the 21st century: New findings and their implications. The American Journal of Psychiatry. 2018;**175**(10):943-950. DOI: 10.1176/appi.ajp.2018.18040383

[24] Leyfer OT, Woodruff-Borden J, Klein-Tasman BP, Fricke JS, Mervis CB. Prevalence of psychiatric disorders in 4 to 16-year-olds with Williams syndrome. American Journal of Medical Genetics. Part B, Neuropsychiatric Genetics. 2006;**141B**(6):615-622. DOI: 10.1002/ajmg.b.30344

[25] Niklasson L, Rasmussen P, Oskarsdóttir S, Gillberg C. Attention deficits in children with 22q.11 deletion syndrome. Developmental Medicine and Child Neurology. 2005;**47**(12):803-807. DOI: 10.1017/S0012162205001702

[26] Vissers LE, Gilissen C, Veltman JA. Genetic studies in intellectual disability and related disorders. Nature Reviews. Genetics. 2016 Jan;**17**(1):9-18. DOI: 10.1038/nrg3999

[27] Chaste P, Roeder K, Devlin B. The Yin and Yang of autism genetics: How rare de novo and common variations affect liability. Annual Review of Genomics and Human Genetics. 2017;**18**:167-187. DOI: 10.1146/annurev-genom-083115-022647

[28] Kirov G, Pocklington AJ, Holmans P, Ivanov D, Ikeda M, Ruderfer D, et al. De novo CNV analysis implicates specific abnormalities of postsynaptic signalling complexes in the pathogenesis of schizophrenia. Molecular Psychiatry. 2012;**17**(2):142-153. DOI: 10.1038/mp.2011.154

[29] Martin J, Hosking G, Wadon M, Agha SS, Langley K, Rees E, et al. A brief report: de novo copy number variants in children with attention deficit hyperactivity disorder. Translational Psychiatry. 2020;**10**(1):135. DOI: 10.1038/s41398-020-0821-y

[30] Lionel AC, Crosbie J, Barbosa N, Goodale T, Thiruvahindrapuram B, Rickaby J, et al. Rare copy number variation discovery and cross-disorder comparisons identify risk genes for ADHD. Science Translational Medicine. 2011;**3**(95):95ra75. DOI: 10.1126/scitranslmed.3002464

[31] Schneider M, Debbané M, Bassett AS, Chow EW, Fung WL, van den Bree M, et al. International Consortium on brain and behavior in 22q11.2 deletion syndrome: Psychiatric disorders from childhood to adulthood in 22q11.2 deletion syndrome: Results from the international Consortium on brain and behavior in 22q11.2 deletion syndrome. The American Journal of Psychiatry. 2014;**171**(6):627-639. DOI: 10.1176/appi.ajp.2013.13070864

[32] Ben-Shachar S, Lanpher B, German JR, Qasaymeh M, Potocki L, Nagamani SC, et al. Microdeletion 15q13.3: A locus with incomplete penetrance for autism, mental retardation, and psychiatric disorders. Journal of Medical Genetics. 2009;**46**(6):382-388. DOI: 10.1136/jmg.2008.064378

[33] Lowther C, Costain G, Stavropoulos DJ, Melvin R, Silversides CK, Andrade DM, et al. Delineating the 15q13.3 microdeletion phenotype: A case series and comprehensive review of the literature. Genetics in Medicine. 2015;**17**(2):149-157. DOI: 10.1038/gim.2014.83

[34] Williams NM, Zaharieva I, Martin A, Langley K, Mantripragada K,

Fossdal R, et al. Rare chromosomal deletions and duplications in attention-deficit hyperactivity disorder: A genome-wide analysis. Lancet. 2010;**376**(9750):1401-1408. DOI: 10.1016/S0140-6736(10)61109-9

[35] Sánchez-Mora C, Ramos-Quiroga JA, Bosch R, Corrales M, Garcia-Martínez I, Nogueira M, et al. Case-control genome-wide association study of persistent attention-deficit hyperactivity disorder identifies FBXO33 as a novel susceptibility gene for the disorder. Neuropsychopharmacology. 2015;**40**(4):915-926. DOI: 10.1038/npp.2014.267

[36] Elia J, Glessner JT, Wang K, Takahashi N, Shtir CJ, Hadley D, et al. Genome-wide copy number variation study associates metabotropic glutamate receptor gene networks with attention deficit hyperactivity disorder. Nature Genetics. 2011;**44**(1):78-84. DOI: 10.1038/ng.1013

[37] Lima Lde A, Feio-dos-Santos AC, Belangero SI, Gadelha A, Bressan RA, Salum GA, et al. An integrative approach to investigate the respective roles of single-nucleotide variants and copy-number variants in attention-deficit/hyperactivity disorder. Scientific Reports. 2016;**6**:22851. DOI: 10.1038/srep22851

[38] Lesch KP, Selch S, Renner TJ, Jacob C, Nguyen TT, Hahn T, et al. Genome-wide copy number variation analysis in attention-deficit/hyperactivity disorder: Association with neuropeptide Y gene dosage in an extended pedigree. Molecular Psychiatry. 2011;**16**(5):491-503. DOI: 10.1038/mp.2010.29

[39] Yang L, Neale BM, Liu L, Lee SH, Wray NR, Ji N, et al. Psychiatric GWAS Consortium: ADHD subgroup: Polygenic transmission and complex neuro developmental network for attention deficit hyperactivity disorder: Genome-wide association study of both common and rare variants. American Journal of Medical Genetics. Part B, Neuropsychiatric Genetics. 2013;**162B**(5):419-430. DOI: 10.1002/ajmg.b.32169

[40] Akutagava-Martins GC, Rohde LA, Hutz MH. Genetics of attention-deficit/hyperactivity disorder: An update. Expert Review of Neurotherapeutics. 2016;**16**(2):145-156. DOI: 10.1586/14737175.2016.1130626

[41] Deciphering Developmental Disorders Study: Prevalence and architecture of de novo mutations in developmental disorders. Nature 2017;542(7642):433-438. doi: 10.1038/nature21062

[42] Willsey AJ, Fernandez TV, Yu D, King RA, Dietrich A, Xing J, Sanders SJ, Mandell JD, Huang AY, Richer P, Smith L, Dong S, Samocha KE; Tourette International Collaborative Genetics (TIC Genetics); Tourette Syndrome Association International Consortium for Genetics (TSAICG), Neale BM, Coppola G, Mathews CA, Tischfield JA, Scharf JM, State MW, Heiman GA: De Novo Coding Variants Are Strongly Associated with Tourette Disorder. Neuron. 2017;94(3):486-499.e9. doi:10.1016/j.neuron.2017.04.024

[43] Huang AY, Yu D, Davis LK, Sul JH, Tsetsos F, Ramensky V, et al. Gilles de la Tourette Syndrome GWAS Replication Initiative (GGRI): Rare Copy Number Variants in NRXN1 and CNTN6 Increase Risk for Tourette Syndrome. Neuron. 2017;**94**(6):1101-1111.e7. DOI: 10.1016/j.neuron.2017.06.010

[44] Rommelse NN, Franke B, Geurts HM, Hartman CA, Buitelaar JK. Shared heritability of attention-deficit/hyperactivity disorder and autism spectrum disorder. European Child & Adolescent Psychiatry. 2010;**19**(3):281-295. DOI: 10.1007/s00787-010-0092-x

[45] Lichtenstein P, Carlström E, Råstam M, Gillberg C, Anckarsäter H. The genetics of autism spectrum disorders and related neuropsychiatric disorders in childhood. The American Journal of Psychiatry. 2010;**167**(11):1357-1363. DOI: 10.1176/appi.ajp.2010.10020223

[46] Martin J, Cooper M, Hamshere ML, Pocklington A, Scherer SW, Kent L, Gill M, Owen MJ, Williams N, O'Donovan MC, Thapar A, Holmans P: Biological overlap of attention-deficit/hyperactivity disorder and autism spectrum disorder: evidence from copy number variants. J Am Acad Child Adolesc Psychiatry. 2014;53(7):761-70.e26. doi: 10.1016/j.jaac.2014.03.004

[47] Harich B, van der Voet M, Klein M, Čížek P, Fenckova M, Schenck A, et al. From rare copy number variants to biological processes in ADHD. The American Journal of Psychiatry. 2020;**177**(9):855-866. DOI: 10.1176/appi.ajp.2020.19090923

[48] Hormozdiari F, Penn O, Borenstein E, Eichler EE. The discovery of integrated gene networks for autism and related disorders. Genome Research. 2015;**25**(1):142-154. DOI: 10.1101/gr.178855.114

[49] Chen W, Zhou K, Sham P, Franke B, Kuntsi J, Campbell D, et al. DSM-IV combined type ADHD shows familial association with sibling trait scores: A sampling strategy for QTL linkage. American Journal of Medical Genetics. Part B, Neuropsychiatric Genetics. 2008;**147B**(8):1450-1460. DOI: 10.1002/ajmg.b.30672

[50] Thapar A, Martin J, Mick E, Arias Vásquez A, Langley K, Scherer SW, et al. Psychiatric gene discoveries shape evidence on ADHD's biology. Molecular Psychiatry. 2016;**21**(9):1202-1207. DOI: 10.1038/mp.2015.163

[51] Kollins SH, McClernon FJ, Fuemmeler BF. Association between smoking and attention-deficit/hyperactivity disorder symptoms in a population-based sample of young adults. Archives of General Psychiatry. 2005;**62**(10):1142-1147. DOI: 10.1001/archpsyc.62.10.1142

[52] Levin ED, Conners CK, Silva D, Hinton SC, Meck WH, March J, et al. Transdermal nicotine effects on attention. Psychopharmacology. 1998;**140**(2):135-141. DOI: 10.1007/s002130050750

[53] D'Souza MS, Markou A. Neuronal mechanisms underlying development of nicotine dependence: Implications for novel smoking-cessation treatments. Addiction Science & Clinical Practice. 2011;**6**(1):4-16

[54] Hollenbeck D, Williams CL, Drazba K, Descartes M, Korf BR, Rutledge SL, et al. Clinical relevance of small copy-number variants in chromosomal microarray clinical testing. Genetics in Medicine. 2017;**19**(4):377-385. DOI: 10.1038/gim.2016.132

Section 2

ADHD Comorbidity and Its Impact on Many Aspects of Development

Chapter 4

Comorbidity in Children and Adolescents with ADHD

Marija Burgić Radmanović and Sanela-Sanja Burgić

Abstract

Attention Deficit Hyperactivity Disorder with or without hyperactivity disorder is a neurobiological disorder that involves the interaction of the neuroanatomical and neurotransmitter systems. It is a developmental disorder of psychomotor skills that is manifested by impaired attention, motor hyperactivity and impulsivity. This disorder is characterized by early onset, the association of hyperactive and poorly coordinated behavior with marked inattention and lack of perseverance in performing tasks; and this behavior occurs in all situations and persists over time. This disorder is inappropriate for the child's developmental age and maladaptive. Disorders of neurotransmitter metabolism in the brain with discrete neurological changes can lead to behavioral difficulties and other psychological problems. Most children and adolescents with Attention Deficit Hyperactivity Disorder have comorbidities, often multiple comorbid conditions in the same person. Comorbidity was observed in both clinical and epidemiological samples. It is estimated that about two-thirds of children with this disorder have at least one other psychiatric disorder diagnosed. Symptoms persist and lead to significant difficulties in the daily functioning of the child, such as school success, social interactions, family and social functioning, etc. Recent studies indicate the presence of various neuroophthalmological disorders in children and adolescents with ADHD. The most common comorbidities in children and adolescents with ADHD that will be covered in this chapter are autism spectrum disorder, mood disorder, anxiety, learning disabilities, conduct disorders, tics disorder and epilepsy.

Keywords: child, adolescent, ADHD, comorbidity, development

1. Introduction

ADHD is a neurobiological disorder that encompasses the specifics of neurotransmitter metabolism brain, and the interaction of the neuroanatomical and neurotransmitter systems. It is a developmental disorder of psychomotor skills that is manifested by impaired attention, motor hyperactivity and impulsivity [1]. Disorders of neurotransmitter metabolism in the brain with discrete neurological changes can lead to behavioral difficulties and other psychological problems. Behavioral disorders, secondary psychological problems, and interaction disorders with mild neurological symptoms may occur with this disorder [2]. To make a diagnosis, the symptoms must be frequent and severe than in children of comparable developmental level, and they must cause significant difficulties in the child's daily functioning [3]. It is a behavioral disorder that makes it difficult for a child to focus on daily requirements and routines. These children and adolescents usually have difficulty organizing, focusing, making realistic plans, and thinking before they do something. The group of authors considers that ADHD is a developmental disorder of lack of behavioral inhibition, which manifests itself as a developmentally inappropriate degree of inattention, excessive activity and impulsivity, and complicates self-regulation and organization of behavior in relation to the future [4]. The main symptoms of ADHD are developmentally inappropriate for the age of the child and these are developmentally inappropriate levels of poor attention, hyperactivity and impulsivity. The degree of intensity of symptoms can vary according to the age of the child. Symptoms are manifested in the form of inattention of the child, the child does not perform its tasks, cannot organize, easily distracted, loses school and other things, "forgetful", avoids prolonged exertion.

The clinical picture in boys and girls differs in some aspects of the symptoms. Boys are more motor hyperactive and girls are more inattentive, as if "dreaming"; and their hyperactivity manifests itself as emotional and verbal (in the form of chatter, crying, etc.).

Data on the frequency of this disorder in developmental age differ depending on the applied methodology, age of the respondents, urban or rural region, number of persons providing data on the child's behavior (only parents, only teachers or both parents and teachers and others). Symptoms of hyperactivity are manifested in such a way that the child fidgets, gets up and leaves the bench, cannot play or do a task in peace, talks a lot, runs and climbs excessively, is always ready to "go" and others. Symptoms of impulsivity in a child are manifested by the child not being able to wait his turn, interrupting others when they speak, giving hasty answers, behaving intrusively and the like. Due to the symptoms, these children achieve poorer success in school, they have difficulties in mastering the school program, although they are most often of normal intellectual potential. Most adolescents who had ADHD as children still have difficulties in schooling, social interactions, and often emotional problems. Some adolescents may show irritability, poor school performance, disorganized learning, and poor communication with peers. ADHD always appears in early development, usually in the preschool period, and is most often noticed when a child starts school. This disorder usually lasts during schooling, and in some it continues into adulthood. Many people may experience improved activity and attention. Children with ADHD are often careless and impulsive so they are prone to accidents and injuries. These children often break the agreed rules and often have disciplinary difficulties. In relationships with adults, children with ADHD are often socially disinhibited, without caution and reserve, reckless behavior. Other children often avoid them, and are considered unpopular among peers, so they are often isolated.

The prevalence of ADHD is between 5 and 7% for children and between 3 and 5% for adults [5]. According to systematic review and meta-analysis, prevalence of ADHD among school-aged children and adolescent vary from 2.2% to 17.8% worldwide [6]. According to epidemiological studies, ADHD in children is thought to continue in 50–80% of cases in adolescence and adulthood. This high prevalence is of concern because this disorder negatively affects all neurodevelopmental areas and the psychosocial interactions of affected individuals. The risk may increase if symptoms such as aggression and irritability or comorbidities, such as behavioral disorders, are present.

In researching this problem, there are certain challenges in estimating the incidence of ADHD, such as are ways to assess ADHD, diagnostic methods, source of information about the disorder, agreement among respondents assessing ADHD symptoms, conducting assessments in one or more settings, age range of respondents, geographical location and characteristics of the community from which respondents originate [5].

Many studies indicate that ADHD is more common in boys [7]. The prevalence in boys and girls varies in different studies, and generally is more likely to be diagnosed and treated in boys than in girls [8]. The ratios from the clinical samples are higher than the ratios from the population samples. Research in this area of developmental psychiatry is extensive with a steady increase in the number of authors and professional literature dealing with this issue.

2. Comorbidity

The term "comorbidity" was introduced into medicine by Feinstein in 1970 to denote those cases in which a particular clinical entity exists simultaneously in a patient during the clinical course of his underlying disease [9]. Psychiatric disorders may coexist with somatic disorders and/or other psychiatric disorders when referring to "psychiatric comorbidity".

Different causes can lead to comorbidities, which can be accidental or the result of a combination of different risk factors; or two disorders may have the same or overlapping risk factors when one disorder causes the other; or there may be a multiform manifestation of one of the two basic disorders when the third - independent – occurs disorder. Due to insufficient knowledge of the etiopathogenesis of psychiatric disorders, modern classification systems (DSM and MKB) apply a descriptive, categorical system that classifies psychiatric symptoms and behaviors into a large number of different diagnoses.

The disadvantage of classification systems is that they poorly recognize the specifics and needs of child and adolescent psychiatry. The diagnostic process in developmental psychiatry is based on descriptive facts that determine the type of disorder, with the use of comorbidities to correct the shortcomings of this diagnostic process and to bring the diagnostic categories closer to the real clinical situation. These specifics are: symptomatic, developmental, environmental and prognostic. In developmental psychiatry, there are specific limitations in the external manifestation of symptoms, as well as in the possibility of insight into the existence of dependent symptoms. In child and adolescent psychiatry, there is the possibility of uneven development of basic developmental lines such as cognitive, emotional and social, especially during early childhood. In childhood, there is a clear dependence on past and current environmental conditions. Their interaction largely determines the manifestation of mental disorder at this age.

ADHD is one of the most common neurodevelopmental disorders in child and adolescent psychiatry and one of the most researched disorders in child psychiatry. Previous research indicates the existence of high comorbidity between ADHD and other psychiatric disorders in childhood. The presence of comorbidities largely depends on: case definition, assessment methodology, and control group. Studies have shown a high comorbidity between ADHD and behavioral disorders in the form of opposition and defiance, depression and anxiety. Some mechanisms for comorbidity include shared risk factors, distinct subtypes and weak causal relationships [10].

A 2015 study by Masi et al. showed more than 2/3 of patients with ADHD have a psychiatric disorder associated. The most common comorbid diagnoses with ADHD during early childhood are oppositional defiant disorder, enuresis and language disorder, and anxiety and tics in the mid-school years. In adolescence are observed mood disorder and substance use disorder. Many children with ADHD have a specific learning disorder [11]. The same study estimates that oppositional defiant disorder is concomitant with ADHD in 25–75% of the cases, conduct disorder about one third of cases, 6–30% of ADHD children have major depression, more than 20% of bipolar disorder co-occur with ADHD; 87% of disruptive mood dysregulation disorder children had ADHD concomitantly; the prevalence of PTSD in children with ADHD is 5.2%; chronic tics disorder with ADHD is 55%; 85% of children with autistic spectrum disorder show a clinical picture of ADHD [11].

Barkley states that 67–80% of children diagnosed with ADHD who have been referred for clinical treatment have at least one more diagnosis, and almost half of them have two diagnoses [5]. Two-thirds of children with ADHD have at least one other psychiatric disorder diagnosed [12].

Some conditions occur more often than others. These are most often the following conditions:

- learning difficulties
- oppositional-defiant behavior
- conductive disorders
- behavioral disorders
- speech-language difficulties
- epilepsy
- mood disorders
- anxiety disorders
- sleep disorders
- tics/Tourette's syndrome
- obsessive–compulsive disorder
- eating disorders

The presence of comorbidities is significant because it complicates the diagnostic process, affects the course, prognosis and therapeutic process. Assessment and support in comorbid disorders are often as important as the assessment and treatment of ADHD symptoms [12].

2.1 Comorbidity with behavioral disorders

Behavioral disorders in developmental age are characterized by persistent and repetitive patterns of dissocial, aggressive, or defiant behavior. These behaviors in their most pronounced form can have criminogenic characteristics and deviate significantly from the socially expected ones according to the age of the child. These disorders are often accompanied by an unfavorable psychosocial environment, unsatisfactory family relationships and school failure. They are more commonly observed in boys than in girls.

Opposition-defiant behavior usually occurs in younger children, who exhibit extremely defiant, provocative, and disobedient behavior, and some children also exhibit aggressive behaviors. Most authors believe that 45–84% of children and adolescents with ADHD also exhibit oppositional-defiant behavior [5]. The

Multimodal Treatment Study of ADHD found that about 62% of preschool children with ADHD and 59% of school children in the sample had oppositional-defiant behavior [5]. It is hypothesized that emotional dysregulation that occurs in children with ADHD may affect the occurrence of comorbidities for oppositional-defiant behavior, anxiety, depression, bipolar disorder, and other conditions, and it has also been observed that these children often have more psychopathology and social problems in the family [5]. These children are also at higher risk of taking various psychoactive substances, rejection from peers, poorer school achievement, rejection and the development of anxiety and depression in adolescence.

Many children with oppositional-defiant behavior also have conductive disorder, which is manifested by recurrent antisocial, aggressive, or defiant behavior. Study by Pliszka included 1035 children and adolescents at a psychiatric clinic and reported that 167 children and adolescents with ADHD were also diagnosed with oppositional defiant or conductive disorder [13]. Research demonstrated that 30–50% children with ADHD fulfill criteria for conduct disorder or oppositional defiant disorder [14]. These children are also at higher risk of substance abuse, antisocial activities, rejection from peers, school failure, anxiety and depression. The families of these children show more psychopathology and social problems.

2.2 Comorbidity with specific learning difficulties

These specific developmental disorders of school abilities include a group of disorders that are characterized by significant difficulties and impairments in mastering school skills, such as reading and arithmetic. These learning disabilities are not a direct result of other disorders such as mental retardation, neurological diseases, uncorrected vision or hearing disorders, or emotional disorders; although they may co-exist with them. Developmental disorders of school ability often exist in comorbidity with ADHD.

These disorders are thought to have arisen from abnormalities in cognitive processing that are mainly the result of some biological dysfunction; and are more common in boys than in girls. These children experience academic failure, often irregular schooling, difficulties in social adjustment and this is more pronounced in the later years of primary school or secondary school.

Specific learning difficulties are more common in people with ADHD than in the general population [15]. A meta-analysis of previous research has concluded that the prevalence is 45% [16]. These children have greater learning difficulties than children who have only specific learning difficulties.

Children with ADHD and specific learning difficulties have a problem processing perceived information, difficulty reproducing words, sentences and letters, auditory discrimination, difficulty reproducing drawings (visual-motor discrimination), stringing letters, decoding letters or words [2]. Children with this comorbidity will have lower academic achievement, poorer grades in school, will drop out of high school more often, and will continue their education after high school less often than their peers without ADHD [5].

2.3 Comorbidity with mood disorders

The main disorder in mood disorders is a change in mood or affect, in the sense of the presence of low mood or excessively good mood. A change in mood is usually accompanied by a change in the overall level of functioning. Most of these disorders show a tendency to recur. The onset of individual episodes is often associated with certain stressful events.

Children and adolescents diagnosed with ADHD often have mood disorders at the same time, most commonly having major depressive disorder, depressive episodes, and bipolar disorder. Arnold et al. conducted a Longitudinal Assessment of Manic Symptoms and concluded that 60% of the sample met the criteria for ADHD, 6.3% met the criteria for bipolar disorder, 16.5% had both ADHD and bipolar disorder. 17.5% do not have either of these two disorders [17]. Otherwise, the results of research in this area are uneven, so in population samples the prevalence is 0–2%, while in clinical samples it is 11–30% [18]. A special problem is the diagnosis, differential diagnosis and treatment in children who have ADHD and mania. ADHD is more common in children, especially in boys, compared with bipolar disorder, which occurs in 1.8% of children and adolescents, and is somewhat more common in boys [19]. Comparing the symptoms of mania and ADHD, a high percentage of grandiosity is noticeable in mania (85%), while in ADHD it is only 6.7%. Elevated mood and bold behaviors occur in a high percentage in mania (87% and 79%, respectively), and in a very low in children with ADHD. Results from regression analyses suggest cognitive predictors of executive functioning impairment in ADHD and mood predictors for inhibition in pediatric bipolar disorder [20].

Comparing the symptoms between these two diseases in childhood, it is noticed that irritability is very pronounced in mania, and occasionally exists in ADHD; euphoria is excessive in mania, and situational in ADHD; children with ADHD have low self-esteem, while mania has a pronounced grandiosity; manic children have a reduced need for sleep, while children with ADHD resist going to bed but then sleep well; children with mania have a rapid flow of thought, while ADHD does not. In comorbidity, treatment preference is given to symptoms of high mood and therapy is primarily focused on mania (mood stabilizers or antipsychotics); while ADHD symptoms are treated secondarily, after mood stabilization.

One of the mood disorders that occurs in child psychiatry is depression. Studies in this area indicate that the prevalence of depression in children with ADHD is 18%, and another 15% had both comorbid anxiety and depressive disorder [21]. The presence of depression worsens the symptoms and functioning of children with ADHD, and also significantly worsens the prognosis and therapeutic process in these children.

Adolescents who have a comorbidity of ADHD and depression have more pronounced difficulties in social functioning, get depression at an earlier age, have a higher rate of suicidal behavior, more frequent recurrence of depressive episodes compared to adolescents who suffer only from depression. Also, these adolescents have more frequent family dysfunction, more frequent conflicts in family relations, they have experienced more negative life events and traumatic experiences compared to adolescents who have only ADHD.

2.4 Comorbidity with anxiety disorders

The prevalence of anxiety disorders in the general pediatric population is between 4% and 20%, while the prevalence of anxiety disorders in children with ADHD is 25% [22]. Clinical and epidemiological studies have shown that one-third of children with ADHD have some of the anxiety disorders at the same time. While some authors believe that there is no statistically significant difference between girls and boys in ADHD comorbidity and anxiety disorder, other authors state that 17.6% of girls and 17.9% of boys have comorbid ADHD disease with anxiety or depressive disorder [8]. Children suffering from anxiety disorder have higher rates of ADHD [5].

2.5 Comorbidity with the autism spectrum disorder (ASD)

Autism spectrum disorder refers to serious developmental disorders with specific patterns of communication and social interactions. These disorders have differences in the specificity and severity of symptoms, age of onset, level of functioning, and forms of social interactions.

Autistic children often have attention problems and information processing problems that lead to social deficits. In clinical samples, it is estimated that about 10% of children tested for ADHD have some comorbid disorder from the autism spectrum disorder [9] characterized by more pronounced hyperactivity and impulsivity. ADHD is diagnosed in the autism spectrum disorder when the symptoms are very pronounced and permanent with the prior exclusion of medical and other psychiatric conditions that may mimic the symptoms of ADHD. In the treatment of ADHD comorbidities with autism spectrum disorder, the symptoms of both disorders must be treated.

2.6 Comorbidity with specific developmental speech and language disorders

In specific developmental disorders of speech and language, there is damage to the normal patterns of speech acquisition from the early stages of development. These disorders are often accompanied by associated problems such as reading difficulties and interpersonal relationships, emotional problems, and behavioral problems.

Some children who have ADHD also have language difficulties, which are present in both receptive and expressive language. There are also difficulties in other language skills. The results of research on the frequency of these comorbid diseases are different. Recent study estimated 50% of children with ADHD have a comorbid language deficit, while 20 to 60% of children with ADHD have one or more learning disabilities or language problems [23]. Study from 2016 identified language impairments in the majority within the ADHD and reading disorder in >40% in children with ADHD [24]. A group of authors concluded in a 2013 study that children with ADHD exhibit various difficulties in pragmatic language [25].

2.7 Comorbidity with epilepsy

Epilepsy is a chronic brain disease characterized by recurrent epileptic seizures, accompanied by various clinical manifestations and laboratory abnormalities. Important features of epilepsy are chronicity and recurrence of excessive paroxysmal discharge of brain neurons that manifest as epileptic seizures.

Studies in children with ADHD have shown a significant risk of developing epilepsy and other seizures in these children. A study by a group of Norwegian authors in 2013 found that children with ADHD had 2.3% risk of epilepsy, which is four times higher than the general prevalence in children of 0.5% [26]. Previous research has also found a significant association between childhood ADHD and the risk of epilepsy. Epilepsy and ADHD are strongly associated although the underlying factors contributing to their co-occurrence remain unclear [27]. The same study suggests that epilepsy and ADHD share less genetic risk factors as compared with other neurodevelopmental disorders.

Children with ADHD often have irregularities in EEG findings, and an increase in frontal-central theta-wave activity is most common [28].

2.8 Comorbidity with sleep disorders

Inorganic sleep disorders can also occur in children of any age. The most common sleep disorder in children is a sleep–wake cycle disorder, i.e. waking up during the night. This is also the most common reason that worries parents and why they seek professional help. The next most common disorder is when the child delays going to bed, cannot fall asleep when put to bed or when constantly asking for parental attention. Other sleep disorders are less common in children.

Children with ADHD often have difficulty sleeping in the form of frequent waking at night, resistance to going to sleep, they need to fall asleep for a long time. Sleep disorders are more likely to occur if children with ADHD also have some anxiety disorder compared to children who have only ADHD [29]. In observational study in a population of children with ADHD, 63% had moderate or severe sleep problems [30].

Parents of children with ADHD also report that children have difficulty sleeping, resist going to bed, sleep shorter, and often wake up at night. Parents describe these children as tired after waking up compared to children without ADHD [31]. Studies investigating event–related potential (ERP) suggest impaired ability in children with ADHD to conserve the brain oscillations phase associated with stimulus processing [32]. Children with ADHD presented more sleep disturbances when compared to children without the diagnosis. These disorders were diverse, yet inconsistent among the surveys [33].

2.9 Comorbidity with tic

Tic is a sudden, fast, involuntary, aimless and repetitive muscle movement, limited to a certain muscle group or accompanied by vocalization, which worsens in stressful situations and disappears during sleep. Tic disorders are divided into transient and chronic motor or vocal and Tourette's syndrome. There is an irresistible need to repeat the action, and its prevention causes tension. Tick disorders are associated with poor self-esteem, problems in the family environment, difficulties at school. Children and adolescents with tics have a number of other problems such as speech or behavior problems, impulsivity, hyperactivity, obsessive compulsive symptoms. The prevalence of transient and simple tics is 20% in the pediatric population, and chronic motor tics and Tourette's syndrome about 3% [34]. Children with ADHD were 4.1 times more likely to have chronic tic disorder at age 7, and 5.9 times more likely at age 10 [35]. Children with ADHD and chronic tic disorder experienced higher rates of peer problems, and poorer quality of life than those with ADHD alone. Episodes of anger and aggression have been reported in children with tic disorders and are likely to contribute to psychosocial stress and low quality of life. It is assumed that aggressive behavior in children with tic disorders is associated with comorbid attention-deficit hyperactivity disorder [36].

2.10 Comorbidity with neuroophthalmological disorders

Ophthalmological examination of children and adolescents with ADHD is part of their evaluation as it is important to rule out underlaying ocular and neurological conditions that may cause behavioral aberrations. Some children with visual impairment may be misdiagnosed as ADHD. These children are not able to see adequately and in result are not able to keep their attention being focused on object of observation. To our knowledge, there are small number of studies investigating the relationship between ADHD and ocular disorders such as amblyopia, hypermetropia, astigmatism, and heterotropia. Children with amblyopia have greater risk of developing ADHD than their counterparts without amblyopia (1,8 times; hazard ratio 1.81; 95% confidence interval 1.59–2.06) with the greatest risk in amblyopic children with deprivation type, followed by strabismic type and refractive type (hazard ratio 2.14; 95% confidence interval 1.56–2.92; hazard ratio 2.09; 95% confidence interval 1.15–3.79; hazard ratio 1.76; 95% confidence interval 1.54–2.02 respectively). Also, amblyopic children with ADHD tend to be diagnosed at younger age than those without amblyopia (median 8.14 vs. 8.45 years; $P = 0.0096$) [37].

Large cross-sectional study on 75,171 children without any intellectual impairment reported greater prevalence of ADHD among children with vision problems ($p < 0.0001$). Children with vision problems were more likely to have been diagnosed with ADHD than those without vision problems (15.6% vs. 8.3%; $p < 0.001$). Children with vision problems were also more likely to have ever been diagnosed with ADHD (18.6% vs. 10.4%; $p < 0.001$) [38].

Another large-scale cross-sectional study on 116,308 children with ADHD reported significant higher prevalence of ocular disorder in children with ADHD compared to children without ADHD: amblyopia (1.6% vs. 0.9%, $p < 0.001$), hypermetropia (2.4% vs. 1.3%, $p < 0.001$), astigmatism (0.2% vs. 0.1%, $p < 0.001$), and heterotropia (1.1% vs. 0.5%, $p < 0.001$) respectively [39].

Recent studies investigated relationship between ADHD and convergence insufficiency as symptoms of convergence insufficiency may overlap with those of ADHD. Within population of children with convergence insufficiency, three-fold greater incidence of ADHD is reported compared to ADHD incidence in general population. Also ADHD population had three-fold greater incidence of convergence insufficiency [40]. Children with ADHD had significant low near point convergence as well [41].

2.11 Treatment of comorbidities

Comorbid diseases often occur in children and adolescents with ADHD. It is estimated that about 66% of ADHD patients have at least one comorbid disorder, and the most common are learning disorders, sleep disorders, oppositional defiant disorder and anxiety disorders [42]. Treating children and adolescents with ADHD who have comorbid conditions is a challenge for clinicians [43].

When it is necessary to include medications in children with ADHD, existing guidelines suggest starting with a stimulant (methylphenidate MPH or amphetamine AMP). If the stimulant does not achieve an effect then an alternative stimulant is used. If stimulants are not effective or cause more severe side effects, we include nonstimulants (atomoxetine, alpha-2 agonists, and antidepressants) [44]. Stimulants have been approved by the Food and Drug Administration (FDA) in the treatment of ADHD, including methylphenidate and dextroamphetamine and amphetamine mixed salts, and these drugs act by blocking the reuptake of dopamine and norepinephrine into neurons. Side effects including insomnia, headache, changes in appetite, weight loss/gain, irritability and tics should be monitored during treatment with stimulants. Stimulants are the first line in treatment. Non-stimulants (atomoxetine, alpha-2 agonists, and antidepressants) are less effective than stimulants. Children with complicated epilepsy may be at greater risk for ADHD, and some antiepileptic medications may contribute to ADHD symptoms. Tricyclic antidepressants have been used in children with ADHD but can lower seizure threshold and should be avoided in patients with epilepsy. Methylphenidate is effective in treating the symptoms of ADHD in children and adolescents with epilepsy, but the effectiveness is less than that seen in children with ADHD without epilepsy [44].

The comorbidity of ADHD with bipolar disorder (BD) may be associated with more severe symptoms, poorer course, and poor outcome of both conditions, and treatment is further complicated if there is substance abuse [45]. The use of stimulants may be contraindicated in the presence of comorbid drug abuse. Atomoxetine may be effective in treating the symptoms of ADHD in patients with bipolar disorder when used in conjunction with mood stabilizers.

In children with ADHD comorbidities and sleep problems, sleep hygiene and cognitive-behavioral psychotherapy are important, and consideration should be given to changing the dosage and formulation of the stimulant. The use of atomoxetine and melatonin are therapeutic alternatives for children with ADHD and more severe sleep problems [46].

Psychopharmacology is the primary treatment for ADHD, and behavioral treatment is used in combination with medication or in children with minimal impairment or when medication is not possible due to contraindications or parents 'refusal to accept medication. Most guidelines recommend a stepwise approach to treatment, beginning with non-drug interventions and then moving to pharmacological treatment in those most severely affected [47]. In large birth cohort study, where a great majority of children with ADHD used medication, only child characteristics were significantly associated with the use of medication [48]. In this study the authors concluded that the small differences between medicated and unmedicated children, might be due to strong established clinical practices where medication is offered as a treatment option, particularly for hyperkinetic conduct disorder in an egalitarian high-income society.

In a large meta-analysis that included 38 individual studies with 5111 participants aged 3 to 18 years, the authors concluded that methylphenidate may improve teacher-reported ADHD symptoms, teacher-reported general behavior, and parent-reported quality of life among children and adolescents diagnosed with ADHD [49].

Treatment of comorbid diseases in children with ADHD should be multimodal, including pharmacological and nonpharmacological interventions. It is important to recognize the presence of comorbid disease in these children because comorbid diseases complicate the diagnostic and therapeutic process, as well as the outcome of the disease.

3. Conclusion

Attention Deficit Hyperactivity Disorder is a neurobiological disorder that involves the interaction of the neuroanatomical and neurotransmitter systems. This disorder is characterized by early onset, the association of hyperactive and poorly coordinated behavior with marked inattention and lack of perseverance in performing tasks; and this behavior occurs in all situations and persists over time. Most children and adolescents with Attention Deficit Hyperactivity Disorder have comorbidities, often multiple comorbid conditions in the same person. It is estimated that about two-thirds of children with this disorder have at least one other psychiatric disorder diagnosed. Symptoms persist and lead to significant difficulties in the daily functioning of the child, such as school success, social interactions, family and social functioning. The presence of comorbidities is significant because it complicates the diagnostic process, affects the course, prognosis and therapeutic process. Assessment and support in comorbid disorders are often as important as the assessment and treatment of ADHD symptoms.

Conflict of interest

The authors declare no conflict of interest.

Author details

Marija Burgić Radmanović[1*] and Sanela-Sanja Burgić[2,3]

1 Department for Child and Adolescent Psychiatry, University Clinical Center of Republic of Srpska, Banja Luka, Bosnia and Herzegovina

2 Eye Clinic, University Clinical Center of Republic of Srpska, Banja Luka, Bosnia and Herzegovina

3 University of Banja Luka, Faculty of Medicine, Banja Luka, Bosnia and Herzegovina

*Address all correspondence to: marija.burgic-radmanovic@med.unibl.org

References

[1] Sadock BJ, Sadock VA, Ruiz P. Kaplan & Sadock's Concise Textbook of Clinical Psychiatry. 4th ed. Philadelphia: LWW; 2017.

[2] Juretić Z, Bujas Petković Z, Ercegović N. Poremećaj pozornosti/hiperkinetski poremećaj u djece i mladeži. Paediatria Croatia. 2011;55:61-67.

[3] Vaida N, Hussain Mattoo N, Madhosh AG. Intelligence among Attention Deficit Hyperactivitiy Disordered (ADHD) Children (Aged 5-9). J Psychology. 2013;4(1):9-12.

[4] Žic Ralić A, Šifner E. Obilježja vršnjačke interakcije i iskustvo vršnjačkog nasilja kod djece i mladih s ADHD-om. Ljetopis socijalnog rada. 2014;21 (3):453-484.

[5] Barkley RA., R.A. Attention-Deficit Hyperactivity Disorder: A Handbook for Diagnosis and Treatment. Fourth edition. The Guilford Press, New York, SAD. 2014:52-74, 116-130, 140-158, 223-298.

[6] Ayano G, Yohannes K, Abraha M. Epidemiology of attention-deficit/hyperactivity disorder (ADHD) in children and adolescents in Africa: a systematic review and meta-analysis. Ann Gen Psychiatry. 2020;21 (19).

[7] Kudek Mirošević J, Opić S. Behaviours typical of ADHD. Odgojne znanosti June 2010;12(1):167-183.

[8] Slobodin O, Davidovitch M. Gender Differences in Objective and Subjective Measures of ADHD Among Clinic-Referred Children. Front Hum Neurosci. 2019;13:441. Published 2019 Dec 13. doi:10.3389/fnhum.2019.0044

[9] Popović-Deušić S. Komorbiditet u psihijatriji razvojne dobi. Psihijat. dan.2011;43(1)1:95-110.

[10] Gnanavel S, Sharma P, Kaushal P, Hussain S. Attention deficit hyperactivity disorder and comorbidity: A review of literature. World J Clin Cases. 2019;7(17):2420-2426. doi:10.12998/wjcc.v7.i17.2420

[11] Masi L, Gignac M. ADHD and Comorbid Disorders in Childhood Psychiatric Problems, Medical Problems, Learning Disorders and Developmental Coordination Disorder. Clinical Psychiatry. Jan 2015. DOI: 10.21767/2471-9854.100005

[12] Juretić Z, Bujas Petković Z, Ercegović N. Poremećaj pozornosti/hiperkinetski poremećaj u djece i mladeži. Paediatria Croatia. 2011;55:61-67.

[13] Pliszka SR. Comorbid psychiatric disorders in children with ADHD. In R. A. Barkley (Ed.), Attention-deficit hyperactivity disorder: A handbook for diagnosis and treatment. The Guilford Press. 2015:140-168.

[14] Gnanavel S, Sharma P, Kaushal P, Hussain S. Attention deficit hyperactivity disorder and comorbidity: A review of literature. World J Clin Cases. 2019 Sep 6;7(17):2420-2426. doi: 10.12998/wjcc.v7.i17.2420.

[15] Sexton C, Gelhorn HL, Bell JA, Classi MP. The co-occurrence of reading disorder and ADHD: epidemiology, treatment, psychosocial impact, and economic burden. J Learn Disabil. Nov-Dec 2012;45(6):538-64.

[16] DuPaul GJ, Gormley MJ, Laracy SD. Comorbidity of LD and ADHD: implicationds of DSM-5 for assessment and treatment. J Learn Disabil. Jan-Feb 2013;46(1):43-51.

[17] Arnold LE, Demeter C, Mount K, Frazier TW, Youngstrom EA, Fristad M, et al. Pediatric bipolar

spectrum disorder and ADHD: comparison and comorbidity in the LAMS clinical sample. Bipolar Disord. 2011;13:509-521.

[18] Pataki C, Carlson GA. The comorbidity of ADHD and bipolar disorder: any less confusion?. Curr Psychiatry Rep. 2013 jul;15(7):372.

[19] Renk K, White R, Lauer BA, McSwiggan M, Puff J, Lowell A. Bipolar disorder in children. Psychiatry J. 2014;2014:928685. doi:10.1155/2014/928685

[20] Geller B, Zimerman B. Prepubertal and early adolescent bipolarity differentiate from ADHD by manic syptoms, grandiose delusions, ultra-rapid or ultradian cycling. J Affect Disord. 1998;51(2):81-9.

[21] Xia W, Shen L, Zhang J. Comorbid anxiety and depression in school-aged children with attention deficit hyperactivity disorder (ADHD) and selfreported symptoms of ADHD, anxiety, and depression among parents of school-aged children with and without ADHD. Shanghai Archives of Psychiatry. 2015 Dec;27(6):356-367. DOI: 10.11919/j.issn.1002-0829.215115.

[22] D'Agati E, Curatolo P, Mazzone L. Comorbidity between ADHD and anxiety disorders across the lifespan. Int J Psychiatry Clin Pract. 2019 Nov;23(4):238-244. doi: 10.1080/13651501.2019.1628277.

[23] Hughes CW, Pickering J, Baker K et al. Differentiating ADHD from oral language difficulties in children: role of movements and effects of stimulant medication. BMC Psychiatry. 2014;14:370. https://doi.org/10.1186/s12888-014-0370-0

[24] Helland WA, Posserud MB, Helland T, Heimann M, Lundervold AJ. Language Impairments in Children With ADHD and in Children With Reading Disorder. J Atten Disord. 2016 Jul;20(7):581-9. doi: 10.1177/1087054712461530.

[25] Staikova E, Gomes H, Tartter V, McCabe A, Halperin JM. Pragmatic deficits and social impairment in children with ADHD. J Child Psychol Psychiatry. 2013;54(12):1275-1283. doi:10.1111/jcpp.12082

[26] Socanski D, Aurlien D, Herigstad A, Thomsen PH, Larsen TK. Epilepsy in a large cohort of children diagnosed with attention deficit/hyperactivity disorders. Seizure. 2013 Oct;22(8):651-5.

[27] Salpekar J. Links Between Epilepsy and ADHD: Time to Focus and Act. Epilepsy Curr. 2018;18(3):160-161. doi:10.5698/1535-7597.18.3.160

[28] Loo SK, Makeig S. Clinical utility of EEG in attention-deficit/hyperactivity disorder: a research update. Neurotherapeutics. 2012 Jul;9(3):569-87.

[29] Accardo AJ, Marcus CL, Leonard MB, Shults J, Meltzer LJ, Elia J. Associations etween psychiatric comorbidities and sleep disturbances in children with Attention-deficit/hyperactivity disorder. J Dev Behav Pediatr. 2012 Feb;33(2):97-105.

[30] Hvolby A. Associations of sleep disturbance with ADHD: implications for treatment. Atten Defic Hyperact Disord. 2015;7(1):1-18. doi:10.1007/s12402-014-0151-0

[31] Becker SP, Pfiffner LJ, Stein MA, Burns GL, McBurnett K. Sleep habits in children with attention-deficit/hyperactivity disorder predominantly inattentive type and associations with comorbid psychopathology symptoms. Sleep Med. 2016 May;21:151-9. doi: 10.1016/j.sleep.2015.11.011.

[32] Baijot S, Cevallos C, Zarka D, et al. EEG Dynamics of a Go/Nogo Task in Children with ADHD. Brain Sci.

2017;7(12):167. Published 2017 Dec 20. doi:10.3390/brainsci7120167

[33] Martins R, Scalco JC, Ferrari Junior GJ, Gerente JGDS, Costa MDL, Beltrame TS. Sleep disturbance in children with attention-deficit hyperactivity disorder: A systematic review. Sleep Sci. 2019;12(4):295-301. doi:10.5935/1984-0063.20190088

[34] Kim S, Greene DJ, Bihun EC et al. Provisional Tic Disorder is not so transient. Sci Rep. 2019;9:3951. https://doi.org/10.1038/s41598-019-40133-4

[35] Poh W, Payne JM, Gulenc A, Efron D. Chronic tic disorders in children with ADHD. Arch Dis Child. 2018 Sep;103(9):847-852. doi: 10.1136/archdischild-2017-314139.

[36] Benaroya-Milshtein N, Shmuel-Baruch S, Apter A et al. Aggressive symptoms in children with tic disorders. Eur Child Adolesc Psychiatry. 2020;29:617-624. https://doi.org/10.1007/s00787-019-01386-6

[37] Su CC, Tsai CY, Tsai TH, Tsai IJ. Incidence and risk of attention-deficit hyperactivity disorder in children with amblyopia: A nationwide cohort study. Clin Exp Ophthalmol. 2019 Mar;47(2):259-264. doi: 10.1111/ceo.13465.

[38] DeCarlo DK, Swanson M, McGwin G, Visscher K, Owsley C. ADHD and Vision Problems in the National Survey of Children's Health. Optom Vis Sci. 2016 May;93(5):459-65. doi: 10.1097/OPX.0000000000000823.

[39] Ho JD, Sheu JJ, Kao YW, Shia BC, Lin HC. Associations between Attention-Deficit/Hyperactivity Disorder and Ocular Abnormalities in Children: A Population-based Study. Ophthalmic Epidemiol. 2020 Jun;27(3):194-199. doi: 10.1080/09286586.2019.1704795.

[40] Granet DB, Gomi CF, Ventura R, Miller-Scholte A. The relationship between convergence insufficiency and ADHD. Strabismus. 2005 Dec;13(4):163-8. doi: 10.1080/09273970500455436.

[41] Ababneh LT, Bashtawi M, Ababneh BF, Mahmoud IH, Rashdan M, Zahran M. Ocular findings in children with attention deficit hyperactivity disorder: A Case-Control study. Ann Med Surg (Lond). 2020 Aug 15;57:303-306. doi: 10.1016/j.amsu.2020.08.005.

[42] Reale L, Bartoli B, Cartabia M, Zanetti M, Costantino MA, Canevini MP, et al. Comorbidity prevalence and treatment outcome in children and adolescents with ADHD. Eur Child Adolesc Psychiatry. 2017 Dec;26(12):1443-1457. doi: 10.1007/s00787-017-1005-z.

[43] Drechsler R, Brem S, Brandeis D, Grünblatt E, Berger G, Walitza S. ADHD: Current Concepts and Treatments in Children and Adolescents. Neuropediatrics. 2020 Oct;51(5):315-335. doi: 10.1055/s-0040-1701658.

[44] Williams AE, Giust JM, Kronenberger WG, Dunn DW. Epilepsy and attention-deficit hyperactivity disorder: links, risks, and challenges. Neuropsychiatr Dis Treat. 2016;12:287-296. doi:10.2147/NDT.S81549

[45] Perugi G, Vannucchi G. The use of stimulants and atomoxetine in adults with comorbid ADHD and bipolar disorder. Expert Opin Pharmacother. 2015;16(14):2193-204. doi: 10.1517/14656566.2015.1079620.

[46] Chamorro M, Lara JP, Insa I, Espadas M, Alda-Diez JA. Evaluacion y tratamiento de los problemas de sueño en niños diagnosticados de trastorno por deficit de atencion/hiperactividad: actualizacion de la evidencia [Evaluation and treatment of sleep problems in children diagnosed with

attention deficit hyperactivity disorder: an update of the evidence]. Rev Neurol. 2017 May 1;64(9):413-421.

[47] Drechsler R, Brem S, Brandeis D, Grünblatt E, Berger G, Walitza S. ADHD: Current Concepts and Treatments in Children and Adolescents. Neuropediatrics. 2020 Oct;51(5):315-335. doi: 10.1055/s-0040-1701658.

[48] Oerbeck B, Furu K, Zeiner P, Aase H, Reichborn-Kjennerud T, Pripp AH, et al. Child and Parental Characteristics of Medication Use for Attention-Deficit/Hyperactivity Disorder. J Child Adolesc Psychopharmacol. 2020 Sep;30(7):456-464. doi: 10.1089/cap.2019.0019.

[49] Storebø OJ, Ramstad E, Krogh HB, Nilausen TD, Skoog M, Holmskov M, et al. Methylphenidate for children and adolescents with attention deficit hyperactivity disorder (ADHD). Cochrane Database Syst Rev. 2015 Nov 25;(11):CD009885. doi: 10.1002/14651858.CD009885.pub2.

Chapter 5

ADHD and Impact on Language

Clay Brites

Abstract

The language problem in ADHD could be expressed in any age, in different intensity levels, that could bring negative effects in all daily activities and learning process, which depends on the right language acquisition during the child's development. Among the most common comorbidities in ADHD, the abnormalities in language result in greater unsatisfactory evolution and many problems in verbal and nonverbal abilities, and even more in academic life, as a result of losses in reading and writing appropriation.

Keywords: comorbitidy language, ADHD, language, cognitive processing, neuropsychological assessment

1. Introduction

The attention deficit hyperactivity disorder (ADHD) is a neurobiological condition, which starts in childhood and youth phase, derived of genetics and external factors, that features an attention, hyperactivity, and impulsivity deficit excess [1]. It hits worldwide an average of 6–10% of children and 2.5–4% of adults [1, 2]. It also causes emotional self-regulation problems, executive impairment, and space and motor disorganization and may cause language problems in 30–40% of the cases [3].

The language problem in ADHD could be expressed in any age, in different intensity levels, that could bring negative effects in all daily activities and learning process, which depends on the right language acquisition during the child's development. Among the most common comorbidities in ADHD, the abnormalities in language result in greater unsatisfactory evolution and many problems in verbal and nonverbal abilities, and even more in academic life, as a result of losses in reading and writing appropriation [4].

Thus, it is essential to understand the facts that interrelate ADHD with the cognitive and language development process, or particularly where and how ADHD neurobiological dysfunctions affect the dynamic of the neural network responsible for the receptive, integrative, and expressive language structure in different child neurodevelopment levels.

2. The neurobiological aspects of ADHD

ADHD leads to emotional and cognitive self-regulation problems, which affect the executive attention and operational memory in the performance of discretionary, routine, and habitual activities. Tasks with no immediate reward which are, at the same time, necessary, priority, and essential for the development of basic abilities and general learning, adding the capacity of self-engage for whole process conclusions [5].

The cause of this disorder is still unknown but is generated by the interaction between genetic and environmental factors (**Table 1**) and by similar epigenetics mechanisms in neuropsychiatry diseases, and they are caused by polygenic inheritances of irregular transmission and are influenced by the environmental and gender predispositions. In the case of ADHD, the predominance is male, in the ratio of 4:1 [6]. So even without a specific cause, these abovementioned data in conjunction with epidemiological evidence provide to the specialists and international consensus a safe outline to the genetic and environmental risk factors for ADHD development (**Table 1**) [7]. The knowledge about these factors contributes for the clinical surveillance during early childhood in order to observe the possibility of the appearance of the first symptoms, adolescence, and adulthood.

The symptoms and cognitive-behavioral changes of ADHD are the results of abnormalities in several neuronal connections, both cortical and subcortical, which can lead to functional impairments in one or more brain regions at the same time. The most affected and described connections mainly involve the anterior cingulate gyrus, prefrontal cortex, amygdala, striatum, and ventral integumentary area, that is, both voluntary and involuntary regions of attention that regulate the intensity and support of the attentional focus [8]. These regions are interconnected by the action of dopaminergic and noradrenergic neurotransmitters, and their deficits also contribute to lowering the attentional functional of ADHD. Added to them are the maturational delays that can gradually occur in these connections during the first years of life and which are observed in many research-based evidences in the functional neuroimaging of the brains of children with ADHD when compared to typical children. The pace of neuronal and connective maturation is slower, erratic, diffuse, or delimited and can emerge clinically at different times in the life cycle, from early childhood to late adolescence [8, 9].

Neuroimaging exams, much more developed today because of the technological advances associated with neuroscientific research, such as functional magnetic resonance imaging (fMRI), are able to analyze the maturational dissonance present in groups with ADHD from a comparative perspective with case controls. There are also brain morphometry, cortical thickness index, diffusion images (tractography), surface measurements of brain areas, gyration index, and geodetic mapping. These methods have shown that ADHD leads to microstructural changes and modifies the proportions between the functional regions of the brain [10, 11].

Genetic factors	Environment factors
High heritability (76%)	Prematurity
Association between twins (80%)	Low birth weight
Carrier parents (85%)	Perinatal complications
Average prevalence in countries (5.2%)	Maternal smoking
Associated with genetic syndromes	Unstable and needy environments
Associated with 20 genetic mutation	Drug use during pregnancy

Table 1.
Genetics and environments risk factors for ADHD clinical features.

Thus, the various changes present in ADHD can be summarized as dis-maturationals, connectives and productive, and abnormal bioavailability of neurotransmitters in the cortical (top-bottom) and subcortical (bottom-up) networks.

3. Neuropsychological and endophenotypical behavioral aspects of ADHD

If we have a different and inefficient brain to process information, the next question would be: In what and how would it be different? In what functional aspects? What neuropsychological deficits are predominantly present in ADHD?

As there are still no specific biological markers, the description and clinical definition of ADHD is based on the *Diagnostic and Statistical Manual of Mental Disorders* (*DSM-5*) criteria (**Figure 1**) on neuropsychological assessments and on the construction, since the early 2000s, of possible candidate profiles to be its endophenotypes [8, 12]. These parameters help to establish the diagnosis and understand its functional deficits.

ADHD can lead to three major functional deficits: (1) executive attention deficit, (2) operational memory problems, and (3) self-engagement in sequential tasks without reward [13].

Executive attention is responsible for the ability to increase the degree of sensitivity, directing the brain perceptions, and persisting in these analyses, being able to verify the details and the most significant information of any task. It includes selective, sustained, alternating, divided, covered, and spatial attention and is able to manage focal points according to time, space, and priorities. It depends on the connection integrity of frontal areas with the anterior and striated (subcortical) cingulate regions.

Operational/working memory is the ability to immediately memorize sequential information to fully accomplish it without forgetting the most important, decisive priority details and those that require data from other axes of knowledge, seeking to align them with those already memorized. It depends on the integrity of frontal regions with amygdala-hippocampus-striatal connections.

Self-engagement in sequential tasks without reward is the "energetic" amount of self-effort and intention undertook to fully and correctly fulfill a specific activity, task, or request without a greater motivation, or which represents a routine, rule, or command by an authority or institution. We can also call it cognitive self-regulation and it depends on connections between regions of the prefrontal cortex with the striatum, ventral regions of the anterior cingulate cortex, amygdala, and ventral tegmental nucleus.

The ADHD patient has a deficit in these three abilities and, therefore, the presentation of its clinical condition and functional difficulties are predominantly concentrated in executive functions, problems in working memory (verbal and nonverbal), difficulties in executive attention, and insufficient surveillance to fulfill correctly activities without immediate attractiveness or pleasure. Even though these characteristics are well defined, there is still no single endophenotypic pattern for ADHD or a neuropsychological profile. However, this evidence is sufficient to better understand the diagnostic approach in clinical suspicion, which evaluation methods to request, and in interdisciplinary evaluations, how to understand the deficits and discrepancies present in each of them and to associate with the main complaints of the child and the child's school.

Thus, in the neuropsychological evaluation, we have to use the instruments that can measure selective and sustained attention, executive functions, verbal and

The diagnostic criteria of the DSM-5 include 9 signs and symptoms of inattention and 9 of hyperactivity and impulsivity. Diagnosis using these criteria requires ≥ 6 signs and symptoms from at least one group. In addition, it is necessary that the symptoms:

- Be present often for ≥ 6 months
- Be more expressive than expected for the child's level of development
- Occur in, at least, 2 situations (for example, home and school)
- Be present before the age of 12 (at least some symptoms)
- Interfere with the functional capacity at home, at school or at work

Inattention symptoms:

- Does not pay attention to details or makes careless mistakes in schoolwork or other activities
- Has difficulty in keeping attention on tasks at school or during games
- Doesn't seem to pay attention when approached directly
- Does not follow instructions and does not complete tasks
- Has difficulty organizing tasks and activities
- Avoid, dislike or is reluctant to engage in tasks that require maintenance of mental effort over a long period of time
- Often loses objects needed for school tasks or activities
- Easily distracted
- Forgetful in daily activities

Symptoms of hyperactivity and impulsivity:

- Moves or twists hands and feet frequently
- Often moves around the room or other places
- Runs and climbs too often when this type of activity is inappropriate
- Has difficulty playing quietly
- Often moves and acts with euphoria
- Tends to talk too much
- Frequently answers questions abruptly, even before they are completed
- Often finds difficulty to wait for his turn
- Often interrupts others or intervenes in other people's talks

The predominant inattention type diagnosis requires ≥6 signs and symptoms of inattention. The diagnosis of the hyperactive/impulsive type requires ≥ 6 signs and symptoms of hyperactivity and impulsivity. The combined type diagnosis requires ≥ 6 signs and symptoms for each criterion of inattention and hyperactivity/impulsivity.

Figure 1.
ADHD DSM-5 criteria. Source: Refs. [18, 19].

nonverbal working memory, reaction time, and cognitive flexibility. Furthermore, correlate these assessed skills with the behavior of the assessed person during the exam, their reactions, avoidances, profile of behavioral responses to failure and test prolongation, etc. The description of these behaviors should be part of the feedback for the specialized team and will be useful for the conclusions.

4. The impact of ADHD on language neurodevelopment in childhood and school

After it all, and the language? The child's learning, from a young age, in the early years, depends on several factors and, neurobiologically, in his first contact with the world, he needs his sensory and perceptual functions. Vision, hearing, touch, etc. and its perceptual centers in the brain added to the qualitative perceptual functions as well, such as attention and memory, to correctly absorb and fix the selected stimuli in the brain. Language, in this context, results from its innate abilities (presence of a network and integral structure for the language) and the internalization of the "languages" perceived around it. Little is known yet whether ADHD affects more innate or acquired language, but in several comparative studies associating both conditions, it appears that ADHD influences the appearance of language disorders (LDs) much more than the opposite [14, 15]. There are sufficient data demonstrating that, in groups of children with LD, there are proportionally fewer children with ADHD than when evaluating groups of ADHD seeking to verify the presence of LD [16].

The adequate construction and the full development of language structuring processes in childhood depend heavily on attentional, executive, and working memory processes. The union of all these factors in the construction of language can be understood by several psychological theories and theoretical constructs, but it is well summarized in the **phonological buffer** [15, 17, 18]. In language science, the phonological buffer is a neurobiological and cognitive mechanism of language composed of skills that align and influence each other as a dynamics of weights and balances for the perception, memorization, and integration of linguistic sensory stimuli contributing to the development and consolidation, in memory, of processes associated with language structures in a coherent way. Consolidated, this same buffer triggers the emergence of previously selected and memorized phonological data to be used for a given expressive activity in an organized and sequential manner (speaking, reading, writing, etc.).

The skills that make up the buffer are executive attention, working memory, and phonological awareness (**Figure 2**). Among the three, the first two are functions specifically associated with ADHD. In ADHD, both are deficient, unstable, and functionally oscillating and end up negatively influencing the development of speech and language in the early years of life, which are skills that depend on phonological awareness and therefore affect the cognitive processes of language.

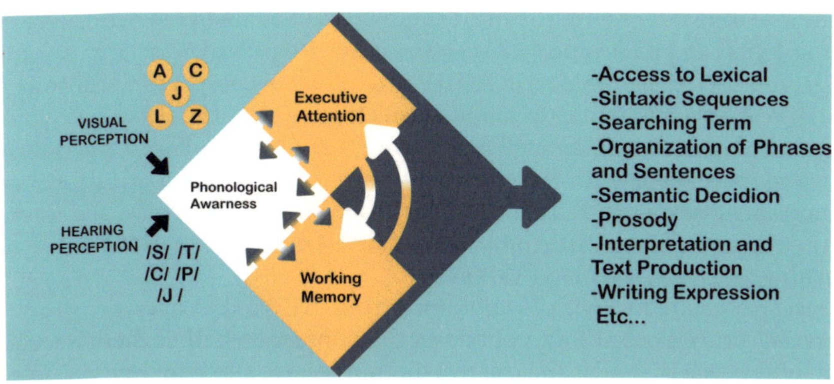

Figure 2.
Interrelation among executive attention, working memory, and phonological awareness to building reading and writing.

In this context, it seems that the selective and sustained attentional deficit would be the main center of disfunction. Attention selectively focuses on one aspect of information and excludes the other. The child who is learning the language from an early age must be able to selectively focus on relevant linguistic information and naturally ignore irrelevant information. He/she must sustain this focus to form an association between an object and a label in the word learning process. When the input source of the language or object changes, the child must also be able to draw attention away to avoid losing relevant information. As language develops, he/she must be able to attend linguistic sequences and social routines for the development of grammatical and pragmatic skills. If he/she cannot do this, whether due to attention deficits or early language problems, the process of language acquisition and consolidation will be fragmented and deficient.

There are also other factors that associate ADHD with language from a genetic and developmental point of view. Children with ADHD may have, in up to 40% of cases, speech development delays because it can affect the perception of sounds during the speech of his peers and caregivers, generate joint problems, and increase chance of stuttering; and by forming phonemes and syllable junction, it is possible to observe a greater slowness in syllabic awareness in these patients [19]. This means the disorder affects attention, motor control (inhibitory and rhythm), and working memory, eventually leading the referred gaps in the evolution of the articulatory and phonological organization.

Another factor described would be the presence of mutations and other genetic abnormalities between both conditions, which would lead to the transmission of their deficits present in the parent(s) to their children. And, finally, the separated association of both conditions that were generated in the same child without one being incidental to the other, but both sharing dysfunctions in specific areas in their interaction, participating in reading and writing language-related functions and language structure [20].

5. Aspects of language influenced by ADHD

Several publications and researches show language alterations in ADHD patients [21]. There is still a need for greater research about the genetic or environmental factors involved. Some evidence describing genes that appear to be at the interface of both conditions already exists, such as FOX2 and CNTNAP2 [22]. But they still lack models that really demonstrate the solid link between them, what kind of comorbidity is included, and what genetic relationships exist (and, specifically, with which genes or mutations). For now, the most common studies are based on relative risk measures (RRs) and odds ratio (OR), and in these, they observe risks of two to six times greater language problems in ADHD groups when compared to controls [19].

ADHD can affect four axes of language in childhood and adolescence: (1) delays in speech acquisition and language structuring (mainly articulatory, phonological, lexical, and morphosyntactical but also, in a second plane, pragmatical); (2) hearing processing disorders; (3) abnormalities in speech (speech, voice, and fluency); and (4) deficits in the linguistic processes involved in the appropriation of reading and writing and math learning (**Table 2**).

In research conducted with 76 children with ADHD and an average age of 11 years old, Bruce e cols. (2006) observed that more than half of them were accompanied by a speech therapist and the rest did not receive any intervention. The results showed that most children had problems in pragmatic language, language comprehension with greater receptive communication deficits and delays, and learning gaps in reading and writing. In this same work, cognitive tests were carried

Axes affected in speech therapy	ADHD effects
Delays in acquiring speech and language during development	Delay in speech acquisition, articulatory errors, memory deficit, and phonological manipulation, problems with rhythm and self-control to speak
Disorders in auditory processing	Deficits in integration, temporality, and association of sounds
Abnormalities in speech	A deficit in pragmatic language and in the perception of prosody during the speech, disrespect to the shifts of conversation, loss of significant moments to understand the intention of the speech, disorganization in the sequence of who will speak, frequent forgetfulness, and long-winded speech
Deficits in the language of reading and writing	Slowness in literacy, delayed processing and spelling engine, poverty in the interpretation and production of texts, spatial trouble remembering quotes and locations in terms of text, and little memorization of facts, concepts, rules that make up the reading and writing

Table 2.
Four axes of language in childhood and adolescence affected for ADHD.

out and the evidence showed that the pragmatic losses were due to the inattention and impulsive behavior of ADHD [23]. There are at least seven ADHD symptoms present in the *DSM-5*, which are indicative of problems associated with communication and language: (1) does not seem to hear when talking directly to him/her; (2) difficulty in carefully following instructions; (3) rush to answer before the questions are even finished; (4) interrupts or intrudes on the conversation of others; (5) difficulty in waiting for dialog shifts; (6) speaks excessively and without self-control; and (7) difficulty in playing silently. Such symptoms have a major negative influence on the construction of communication skills, which can be consolidated during child development and adolescence and remain altered throughout life [2].

Besides, the existence of speech delay, articulatory problems, and stutter are relatively frequent in ADHD. Researches show that 25–40% of the cases suffer from such alterations and that indicates possible harm in complex acquisition with aging until it becomes predisposed comorbidity with dyslexia [24]. Many children with ADHD need speech therapy in their early ages of life, and a great part of them keep the therapy until the beginning of school and literacy years, but demonstrations show that with early intervention, the prognostic can get much better [25]. Pieces of evidence show larger deficits in the phonological and articulatory abilities, semantic structure, vocabulary repertoire, reading comprehension, and pragmatic process during dialogs and discursive abilities [26, 27].

The hearing processing is a set of specific and nonspecific skills associated with the set of skills necessary for an adequate perception, integration, and interpretation of what is heard in the most diverse environments. ADHD, due to its characteristics, especially affects the nonspecific skills necessary for auditory processing: the integrative, temporal, and organizational aspects of auditory discrimination. Almost 50% of cases of auditory processing disorders have comorbid symptoms of ADHD and their treatment requires intervention in both for good results to occur [28, 29].

Regarding discursive skills, several changes are observed in people with ADHD. Problems in sustained attention, impulsiveness to conclude and accelerate the discursive times and attentional lack of control, and seeming not to hear the interlocutor make these patients have greater difficulty in applying the right words and expressions at the right time and with plausible intentionality. Through it away occurs both to listening and delivering speeches and, especially, in the consistent persistence of the records heard, they show sudden and erratic self-distractions, little perception for moments of exclamations and tangential comments, hum and make strange noises during the process, enters with new topics decontextualized, and have little sensitivity to perceive commotions during the speech [2]. These difficulties can lead to great losses in the classroom, in lectures, in the coordination of speeches during a comment, and in the correct and strict understanding of a dialog or a recommendation or even "scolding" or warnings from your parents or caregivers. Perhaps, this explains why these patients tend to repeat the same mistakes or do not understand small insinuations or messages contained in the speeches that they hear and receive severe and repeated criticisms in social relations for this.

The significant problems and deficits observed in the processes of learning to read and write and, even later, in the literacy phase and in the already consolidated phase of the acquisition of these skills in these patients are varied and numerous—and today well described—in the scientific literature. People with ADHD have delays and gaps in the process of acquiring and appropriating basic skills for learning to read and write in up to 30–40% of cases. We see little memorization of graphic and phonemic symbols, difficulty in joining letters, and graphophonemic decoding. They usually forget much of what they saw or heard in class and can evolve greater irregularity so that they will acquire the proper fluency and automatic word recognition, sentences negatively affecting the ability to interpret, assimilate statements, and produce texts coherently. They may have more difficulty in organizing the words and phrases sequentially and "lose themselves" in the cohesion of the set of information they write in addition to often not being able to remember all the significant details to clarify an argument in writing.

Not being able to remember orthographic rules or perceive prosodic circumstances in the text to properly apply punctuation or paragraphs are constant in ADHD and can damage the semantic-pragmatic nexus. The longer and subliminal the writings, the greater the difficulties in textual praxis and the subsequent errors. Not to mention the problems of graphomotor coordination generated by the problems of rhythm, persistence, and inhibiting self-control of manual writing mobility, which in addition to deteriorating handwriting, leads to early tiredness, pain in the limb, and aversion/displeasure toward writing. They do not even take care of their writing tools because they lose, break, and play more with them in their hands. By making use of them at the time of class, they confusingly drop, destroy, and barely manage to stay at your desk during the class period. Furthermore, as they usually strain to perform in a less productive/in-depth manner than their colleagues, their text ends elementary, without details, abbreviated, saving words and, even so, they think what they have done is great and "enough"; but, actually, it had resulted in an insufficient work that is poorly done and that had to be corrected. Persistent, recurring delays lead to a progressive inadequate acquisition of skills and many of these young people progress to learning disorders [19].

All of this evidence can help to understand why ADHD patients act socially more with their hands (by actions) than with their eyes and mouth (by structuring words and arguments) and then being less assertive, wordy, and emotionally loosely organized in social interaction. Not to mention the significant losses in school performance, poor interpretation of statements, and low self-esteem for academic processes. The risk of school failures and dropouts is four times higher in these patients and reduces the chance of completing and receiving a university degree by up to eight times [30, 31].

Finally, the knowledge about these changes by health and education professionals is very important because the effects on the global development of the child's language will lead to a negative, progressive impact in all related areas. The severe appearance of gaps in school learning, in the understanding of verbal and nonverbal processes of social communication, and the emotional and affective relationships that depend on language skills can lead to subjective problems in the patient and in family dynamics with different impacts throughout his life.

6. ADHD and language: The role of speech therapy

In the face of all the observations and the aforementioned evidence, the hearing care professional should be prepared to evaluate these children. Delays in speech and language acquisition should always suggest the possibility of ADHD as well as the presence of quantitative and qualitative deficits in BP, speech skills, and reading and writing, depending on the chronological age. However, studies and publications on ADHD and aspects related to language around the world still lack, except on the area of reading, which is the only one with more robust studies [32].

There is still no protocol or consensual or systematic recommendations on how the speech therapist can act in this area. However, there are articles and publications that can help this professional to create a basic protocol to better direct their work and to assist in a complementary, more refined, and objective way for the interdisciplinary team in order to better conclude the diagnosis and more broadly direct future strategies' therapeutic [32, 33].

Even so, some recommendations can help, right now, to improve the procedures of speech therapy assessment in ADHD:

1. Knowing deeply the signs and symptoms of ADHD.

2. Knowing how to correlate the neurobiology and neuropsychology of ADHD with speech therapy assessment.

3. Track in the child's neurodevelopment early signs of ADHD and possible effects of ADHD on the child's speech and language.

Test name	Age	Domains evaluated
Clinical evaluation of language fundamentals—4	5–21 years	Formulation of sentences, the definition of words, and their classes and semantics
Test of language development primary	4–9 years	Semantics and grammar, reception and expression, and general language skills
Communication abilities diagnostic test	3–9 years	Varied tests for syntax, semantics, and pragmatics during stories, games, and conversations
Language processing test 3: Elementary	5–11 years	Association tasks, categorization, similarities/differences, and multiple meanings and attributes
Children's communication checklist-2	4–16 years	Evaluates verbal and nonverbal social communication
Assessment of comprehension and expression	6–11 years	Understanding sentences, inferences, nonliteral language, and use of narratives
Test of language competence	5–18 years	Ambiguous sentences, comprehension, inferences, and figurative language
Test of pragmatic language	8–18 years	Pragmatic language
Test of attention, executive, and language functions	Under 5 years	Translated available tests, validated in neuropsychology and speech therapy

Table 3.
Instruments in speech therapy for language assessment in ADHD.

4. Knowing more clinically the signs of impaired reading and writing that may be associated with language problems or ADHD.

5. Interpreting the BP test while considering the nonspecific factors that may be negatively influencing the results.

6. Seeking consensus, new publications, and speech therapy forums or congresses that will systematize instruments to be used in the assessment of these children (instruments in speech therapy, even a foreign language, can help a lot) (**Table 3**) [21].

7. Final considerations

Knowing the aspects of ADHD related to the development, structuring and school management of language is essential for undertaking an adequate assessment of these patients during and after the diagnostic process. During, in order to decisively contribute to speech therapy data in the confirmation of a further condition without definitive biomarkers. After, in order to delineate with the results the treatment needs that may involve the speech therapist, who has the role of intensively intervening in deficits that are not within the competence of the school or family but should be corrected by the specialist in order to provide a more favorable and persevering school performance.

Author details

Clay Brites
Neurosaber Institute, Londrina, Paraná, Brazil

*Address all correspondence to: claybrites@gmail.com

References

[1] Polanczyk G, Rodhe LA. Epidemiology of attention-deficit/hyperactivity disorder across the lifespan. Current Opinion in Psychiatry. 2007;**20**(4):386-392

[2] Tannock R. Transtornos da linguagem e da saúde mental: o caso do TDAH. Convergência: Comunicação interdisciplinar. 2004;**2005**:45-53

[3] Rohde LA, Buitelaar JK, Gerlach M, Faraone SV. The World Federation of ADHD Guide. Porto Alegre: Artmed; 2019

[4] Ciasca SM, Rodrigues SD, Salgado CA. Transtorno de Déficit de Atenção e Hiperatividade (TDAH). 1st ed. Porto Alegre: Revinter; 2010

[5] Brites C, Sergeant JA. Transtornos do Déficit de Atenção e Hiperatividade e os Transtornos de Aprendizagem à Luz do Modelo Cognitivo-Energético. In: Ciasca SM, Rodrigues SD, Salgado-Azoni CA, Lima RF, editors. Transtornos de Aprendizagem: Neurociência e interdisciplinaridade. Ribeirão Preto: Book Toy; 2015

[6] Nigg JT, Nikolas M, Burt SA. Measured gene-by-environment interaction in relation to ADHD. Journal of the American Academy of Child and Adolescent Psychiatry. 2010;**49**(9):863-873

[7] Banerjee TD, Middleton F, Faraone SV. Fatores de risco ambientais para transtorno de déficit de atenção e hiperatividade. Acta Paediatrica. 2007;**96**(9):1269-1274

[8] Montes LGA, Alcántara HP, García RBM, De La Torre LB, Acosta DA, Duarte MG. Brain cortical thickness: Age, sex and clinical correlations. Journal of Attention Disorders. 2012;**17**(8):641-654

[9] Shaw P, Eckstrand K, Sharp W, Blumenthal J, Lerch JP, Greenstein D, et al. Attention-deficit/hyperactivity disorder is characterized by a delay in cortical maturation. Proceedings of the National Academy of Sciences of the United States of America. 2007;**104**:19649-19654

[10] Rubia K. Cognitive neuroscience of attention deficit hyperactivity disorder (ADHD) and its clinical translation. Frontiers in Human Neuroscience. 2018;**12**:100. DOI: 10.3389/fnhum.2018.00100

[11] Kasparek T, Theiner P, Filova A. Neurobiology of ADHD from childhood to adulthood: Findings of imaging methods. Journal of Attention Disorders. 2015 Nov;**19**(11):931-943

[12] American Psychiatric Association. Diagnostic and Statistical Manual of Mental Disorders: DSM-5. 5th ed. Washington: American Psychiatric Association; 2013

[13] Brites C. Neuropsicologia no TDAH: aspectos clínicos e diagnósticos. In: Machado AC, Bello SF, Borges KK, editors. Neuropsicologia e Aprendizagem. 2nd ed. Ribeirão Preto: Book Toy; 2018

[14] Mueller KL, Tomblin JB. Examining the comorbidity of language disorders and ADHD. Topics in Language Disorders. 2012;**32**(3):228-246

[15] Guardiano M, Candeias L, Guimarães JE, Viana V, Almeida P. Avaliação do processamento fonológico e da compreensão em crianças com PHDA. Psicologia, Saúde & Doenças. 2013;**14**(3):420-436

[16] Beitchman JH, Wilson B, Johnson C, Atkinson L, Young AR, Adlaf E, et al. Fourteen-year follow-up of speech/language-impaired and control children: Psychiatric outcome. Journal

of the American Academy of Child and Adolescent Psychiatry. 2001;**40**(1):75-82

[17] Dick MJ, Piek JP. Developmental delays in children with ADHD. Journal of Attention Disorders. 2014;**18**(5):466-478

[18] Rodrigues A, Befi-Lopes DM. Memória operacional fonológica e suas relações com o desenvolvimento da linguagem infantil. Pro-Fono Revista de Atualização Científica. 2009;**21**(1):63-68

[19] Dorneles BV, Corso LV, Costa AC, Pisacco NMT, Sperafico YLC, Rohde LA. Impacto do DSM-5 no Diagnóstico de Transtornos de Aprendizagem em Crianças e Adolescentes com TDAH: Um Estudo de Prevalência. Psicologia: Reflexão e Crítica;**27**(4):759-767

[20] Bruce B, Thernlund G, Nettelbladt U. ADHD and language impairment: A study of the parent questionnaire FTF (Five to Fifteen). European Child & Adolescent Psychiatry. 2006;**15**:52-60. DOI: 10.1007/s00787-006-0508-9

[21] Tannock R. ADHD and communication disorders. In: Banaschewski T, Coghill D, Zuddas A, editors. Oxford Textbook of ADHD. Glasgow: Oxford University Press; 2018

[22] Vernes SC, Newbury DF, Abrahams BS, Winchester L, Nicod Groszer M, et al. A functional genetic link between distinct developmental language disorders. The New England Journal of Medicine. 2008;**359**:2337-2345

[23] McInnes A, Humphries T, Hogg-Johnson S, Tannock R. Listening comprehension and working memory are impaired in attention-deficit hyperactivity disorder irrespective of language impairment. Journal of Abnormal Child Psychology. 2003;**31**(4):427-443

[24] Boada R, Willcutt E, Pennington BF. Understanding the comorbidity between dyslexia and attention-deficit/hyperactivity disorder. Topics in Language Disorders. 2012;**32**(3):264-284

[25] Oliveira MCV, Pessoa LF, Alves HVD. Linguagem, Funções Executivas e Técnicas de Mapeamento Cerebral nos Primeiros Anos de Vida: Uma Revisão. Estudos e Pesquisas em Psicologia. 2018;**18**(1):341-360

[26] Purvis KL, Tannock R. Language abilities in children with attention deficit hyperactivity disorder, reading disabilities, and normal controls. Journal of Abnormal Child Psychology. 1997;**25**(2):133-144

[27] Barini NS, Hage SRV. Vocabulário e compreensão verbal de escolares com TDAH. CoDAS. 2015;**27**(5):446-451

[28] Rangel DI. Estratégias educacionais como ação mediadora: associação entre distúrbio do processamento auditivo e TDAH. 2008 Tese (Doutorado em Educação) – PUCRS, Porto Alegre; 2008

[29] Cavadas M, Pereira LD, Mattos P. Efeito do metilfenidato no processamento auditivo em crianças e adolescentes com TDAH. Arquivos de Neuro-Psiquiatria. 2007;**65**(1):138-143

[30] Mattos P, Rohde LA. Princípios e práticas em TDAH. Porto Alegre: Artmed; 2016

[31] Kent KM, Pelham M Jr, Molina BSG, Sibley MH, Waschbusch DA, Yu J, et al. The academic experience of male high school students with ADHD. Journal of Abnormal Child Psychology. 2011;**39**(3):451-462

[32] Machado-Nascimento N, Kummer AM, Lemos SMA. Alterações Fonoaudiológicas no Transtorno de

Déficit de Atenção e Hiperatividade: revisão sistemática de literatura. CoDAS. 2016;**28**(6):833-842

[33] Oram J, Fine J, Okamoto C, Tannock R. Assessing the language of children with attention deficit hyperactivity disorder. American Journal of Speech-Language Pathology. 1999;**8**:72-80

Chapter 6

Adult Attention-Deficit/ Hyperactivity Disorder and Substance Use Disorder: A Systematic Review of the Literature

Anja Plemenitaš Ilješ

Abstract

Attention-deficit and hyperactivity disorder (ADHD) often presents with comorbid substance use disorder (SUD). The extant literature on the comorbidity of adult ADHD and SUD was summarized on the etiology, prevalence, diagnosis, and treatment. ADHD is diagnosed in 15–20% of SUD patients, mostly as ADHD with a combined presentation. ADHD and SUD are believed to have shared pathophysiology. ADHD is associated with the majority of dependence diagnoses. A most used screening questionnaire for screening ADHD patients presenting with SUD is the Adult ADHD Self-report Scale (ARSR). Evidence on pharmacological treatment is limited, but new trials support the use of long-acting stimulants as also recommended with a combination of psychotherapy by expert opinion. Given the prevalence of both ADHD and SUD, more research is needed to understand the theoretical and clinical implications of this comorbidity.

Keywords: adult, attention-deficit hyperactivity disorder, comorbidity, substance use disorders, clinical implications

1. Introduction

Attention-deficit and hyperactivity disorder (ADHD) is a neurodevelopmental disorder characterized by persistent symptoms of inattention and/or hyperactivity-impulsivity. There are three subtypes of ADHD, marked by predominantly inattentive symptoms, or by hyperactivity and impulsiveness, either a combination of inattentiveness and hyperactivity [1]. Studies suggest that the prevalence of ADHD among children may be as high as 15.5%, with approximately 20% of cases persisting into adulthood [2, 3]. A lower prevalence of ADHD in adults compared with children is consistent with the age-dependent decline of the disorder, which has been confirmed in a meta-analysis [4]. ADHD is diagnosed twice as often in boys as in girls. Boys with ADHD tend to present with more impulsivity, while girls with ADHD tend to have more inattentiveness [5].

The etiology and pathophysiology of ADHD are incompletely understood. There is evidence of a genetic basis for ADHD and secondary environmental risk factors.

Differences in the dimensions of the frontal lobes, caudate nucleus, and cerebellar vermis have been demonstrated. Neuropsychological studies have demonstrated deficits in executive functioning and alterations in the motivation and reward among individuals with ADHD [6]. There is both empirical and theoretical support for an association between ADHD and SUD. ADHD and SUD are believed to have shared pathophysiology. Dopaminergic dysregulation of the motivational and reward system of the midbrain the basal ganglia and the frontal cortical regions influence executive functions and response inhibition which are key characteristics in both disorders [6, 7].

The essential feature of a substance use disorder (SUD) is a cluster of cognitive, behavioral, and physiological symptoms. This indicates that the individual continues using the substance despite significant substance-related problems. An essential characteristic of SUD is an underlying change in brain circuits. These changes may persist beyond detoxification, particularly in individuals with severe disorders. The behavioral effects of these brain changes may be exhibited in the repeated relapses and intense drug craving when the individuals are exposed to drug-related stimuli. The diagnosis of a SUD is based on a pathological pattern of behaviors related to use of the substance, which includes impaired control over substance use, the consummation of substance in more significant amounts or over a longer period, persistent desire to cut down or regulate substance use, a great deal of time spent in using the substance, craving for the drug, social impairment, risky use of the substance, and pharmacological criteria including tolerance and withdrawal [1].

One of the most frequent co-occurring disorders with adult ADHD is SUD. A meta-analysis reported a prevalence of 15–20% of ADHD in adults diagnosed with SUD (nicotine excluded) [8, 9].

International consensus statement concluded that screening questionnaires such as the Adult ADHD Self-Report Scale (ASRS) are useful in screening patients presenting with SUD followed by in-depth diagnostic assessment if the screener is positive or if the clinician has a strong clinical feeling about the possible presence of ADHD. ADHD and SUD experts agreed that the simultaneous and integrated treatment of ADHD and SUD using a combination of pharmaco- and psychotherapy is recommended [10].

The aim of this study is to summarize extant scientific literature concerning the comorbidity of ADHD and SUD on the etiology, prevalence, diagnosis, and treatment.

2. Methods

Publications on adults with combined ADHD and SUD were included focusing on etiology, prevalence, diagnosis and treatment. PubMed search was performed for articles published between 2010 and 2020 using the terms: adult ADHD, drug abuse, substance use disorder, addiction, and dependence. Publications were limited to articles published in English and were discarded if: they did not include adults; ADHD or SUD was not the primary diagnosis; they were reviews before a meta-analysis; they were personal opinion papers; and they were study protocols. The search was conducted on August 17, 2020.

3. Results

A total of 143 articles were found on initial search and screened on title and abstract. Of these, 68 articles did not discuss a combination of ADHD and SUD specifically. Articles focusing solely on children or discussing other topics were excluded (n = 9) and also those in other languages (n = 7) or they were too old (n = 13). A total of 46 peer-reviewed studies were included for full-text review. Additional five articles were found with cross-referencing cited by authors that had not been found by initial research.

All together 51 articles were focusing either on etiology (n = 6), prevalence and symptom severity (n = 28), screening (n = 4), and treatment (n = 13) of adult ADHD and SUD.

3.1 Etiology

A study exploring childhood trauma exposure in SUD patient with ADHD and control group found higher rates of childhood trauma in ADHD and SUD patients, but not with the persistence of childhood ADHD into adulthood [11]. A familial risk analysis of probands followed from childhood to young adulthood found that SUDs in probands increased the risk for SUDs in relatives irrespective of ADHD status [12].

A large trans-ancestral genome-wide association study (GWAS) of alcohol dependence revealed common genetic underpinnings with ADHD, which indicates shared etiology between the two disorders [13]. Shared genetic susceptibility ADHD and SUD is also reported in Spanish study with polygenic scores based on GWAS [14]. Study on shared genetic contribution of the ADHD and SUD showed significantly increased frequency of the dopamine beta-hydroxylase (DBH) rs2519152 and the opioid receptor mu-1 (OPRM1) risk genotypes rs1799971 [15]. Dutch International Multicenter ADHD Genetics study reported that the serotonin genetic risk score significantly predicted alcohol use severity, but no significant serotonin × dopamine risk score or effect of stimulant medication was found [16]. An Italian study reported that patients with ADHD showed a higher intensity of craving for heroin than patients without ADHD in the absence of withdrawal symptoms. We can conclude on shared neurobiological mechanisms that mutually influence the evolution of both disorders where dopamine dysfunction within various brain circuits may influence impulsivity levels, motivation, inhibitory control, executive functions, and behavior and, consequently, the intensity of craving [17].

A study which analyzed commercial health-care claims from adolescent and adult ADHD patients shows results that receiving ADHD medication is unlikely to be associated with a higher risk of substance-related problems in adolescence or adulthood. Instead, medication was associated with lower concurrent risk of substance-related events and, at least among men, with lower long-term risk of future substance-related events [18].

3.2 Prevalence and symptom severity

Existing evidence shows a prevalence of 15–20% of ADHD in adults diagnosed with SUD [8]. International European study exploring the prevalence of DSM-IV and DSM-5 adult ADHD varied from 5.4 to 32.6%. Prevalence estimates for DSM-5 were slightly higher than for DSM-IV [19]. Another study on inpatients with alcohol dependence showed that ADHD prevalence was 20.5% [20]. Nigerian study observed an ADHD prevalence of 21.5% with the combined subtype being the most prevalent [21].

Adult ADHD was reported to be associated with fewer years of education, earlier initiation of regular tobacco use and more extensive lifetime poly-drug [22], as also with a more severe pattern of cocaine consumption [23]. ADHD in the cocaine-dependent patient was associated with factors such as male gender, age at the start of cocaine use and dependence, the amount of cocaine consumed weekly, increased occupational alteration, alcohol consumption, general psychological discomfort, depressive disorder, and antisocial personality disorder [24]. A large study reported that high rate of ADHD symptoms was found among heroin-dependent patients, particularly those affected by the most severe form of addiction. These individuals had higher rates of unemployment, other comorbid mental health conditions, and heavy tobacco smoking [25]. Another study reported that ADHD in long-term methadone maintenance treatment of patients is characterized by greater addiction severity and more comorbid psychopathology [26]. Mexican study reported that adolescents diagnosed with ADHD were more likely to have problems with use or abuse of or dependence on inhalants, and an elevated prevalence of parental SUDs was found in both the adolescent and adult groups [27].

Data from the National Epidemiologic Survey of Alcohol and Related Conditions (NESARC) on ADHD symptoms (DSM-IV) for the period when they were 17 years old or younger showed that hyperactive-impulsive symptoms were more consistently associated with lifetime substance use and SUD compared to inattentive symptoms [28]. Large American study investigated associations of lifetime hyperactive-impulsive ADHD and inattention ADHD. Both hyperactive-impulsive and inattention group were associated with the majority of dependence diagnoses in a linear pattern, such that each additional symptom was associated with a proportional increase in odds of dependence. Both were uniquely associated with alcohol, nicotine, and polysubstance dependence, but only hyperactive-impulsive ADHD was uniquely associated with dependence on illicit substances [29].

Prospective outcome study reported that adults with childhood ADHD are more susceptible than peers to developing alcohol (adjusted OR 14.38, 95% CI 1.49–138.88) and drug dependence (adjusted OR: 3.48, 95% CI: 1.38–8.79) [30]. A recent Dutch study confirmed this, where results showed that individuals with persistent ADHD were at significantly higher risk of development of SUD relative to healthy controls (OR = 4.56, CI 1.17–17.81). In contrast, levels of SUD in those with remittent ADHD were not different from healthy controls (OR = 1.00, CI: 07–13.02). They concluded that SUD and nicotine dependence are associated with a negative ADHD outcome [31]. Similar results were reported in Italian study where patients with ADHD symptoms and high-dose benzodiazepine dependence showed a significantly larger prevalence of poly-drug abuse than ones without them [32].

A French study reported that a history of ADHD was associated with an earlier onset of addiction, poly-dependence, and borderline personality disorder [33]. An Australian study reported that conduct disorder, rather than ADHD, is the strongest predictor of differences in patterns of drug use severity. The extensive comorbidity of those two highlights the great potential for misattributing drug use risks to ADHD [34]. A Dutch study on opioid-dependent patients found that conduct disorder patients had significantly higher problem severity scores, more frequent comorbid SUD, and more severe psychiatric comorbidity. ADHD was found to increase the risk of psychiatric comorbidity [35]. Another study on British prisoners, on the contrary, show that combined ADHD type is significantly associated with the need for coping as a way of managing primary and comorbid symptoms, but not conduct disorder [36]. Brazilian study also found no difference in drug use or dependence prevalence between ADHD and non-ADHD patients but observed different addiction patterns such as earlier use of cocaine and more severe use of cocaine correlated to earlier contact with cannabis [37]. The longitudinal study followed participants with childhood-limited ADHD and persistent ADHD compared to controls and found that there were no significant group differences in change in rates of substance dependence over time. However, individuals whose ADHD persisted into adulthood were significantly more likely to meet DSM-IV criteria for alcohol, marijuana, and nicotine dependence [38]. An Australian study conducted in drug and alcohol treatment centers reported increased drug dependence complexity and chronicity in treatment-seeking SUD patients who screen positively for ADHD, specifically for amphetamine, alcohol, opiates other than heroin or methadone, and benzodiazepines [39].

A recent large study reported that symptoms of hyperactivity/restlessness and problems with self-concept increased the odds of having a diagnosis of ADHD and that impulsivity mediated the relationship between adult ADHD symptoms and alcohol dependence severity [40]. A Dutch study showed higher levels of motor and cognitive impulsivity in ADHD patients with comorbid cocaine dependence compared to ADHD patients without cocaine dependence and controls [41]. Belgian study also reported higher impulsivity in cocaine-dependent individuals to controls, regardless of whether they have concomitant ADHD or not [42]. Similar was reported by Brazilian study where patients who had ADHD and cocaine dependence had impairments in both cognitive and affective regulation [43]. Another study on cocaine dependence reported that the Barkley's executive dysfunction items showed statistically significant differences between cocaine-dependent patients with ADHD and those patients without ADHD diagnosis [44].

Swiss study reported that patients with probable adult ADHD showed higher craving, more withdrawal and psychiatric symptoms, and rated withdrawal symptoms as more severe than did patients without ADHD symptoms [45]. Hungary study of drug-dependent patients with and without ADHD symptoms reported the highest severity of aggression when the ADHD positive status co-occurred with heroin use, while the lowest severity of aggression was detected when ADHD negative status co-occurred with the use of marijuana. ADHD positive patients showed a marked increase in depression symptoms, suicidal ideation, suicidal attempts, as well as self-injuries associated with suicidal attempts [46]. Study on Scottish prisoners reported that ADHD symptoms were the strongest predictor, followed by alcohol dependence for violent offending. Hence, the authors pointed out the importance to treat drug addiction and ADHD symptoms in order to reduce offending among the most persistent offenders [47]. Taiwan study among heroin-dependent participants entering methadone maintenance treatment showed that ADHD-screened positive patients showed higher depression scores ($p = .003$), and more severe heroin dependence ($p = .006$) [48]. Childhood ADHD was associated with obsessive-compulsive disorder, and both conditions were highly prevalent among former heroin addicts on methadone maintenance treatment [49].

3.3 Screening and diagnosis of ADHD and SUD

ADHD is a common comorbid disorder that is frequently overlooked in adults with SUD. DIVA diagnostic interview is important tool to diagnose ADHD in adult patients. Since it is an interview, it has greater diagnostic power then screening questioners. DIVA-5 is the successor to DIVA 2.0, the structured Diagnostic Interview for Adult ADHD, and is based on the criteria for ADHD in DSM-5 [50]. A most used screening questionnaire for screening ADHD patients presenting with SUD is the ASRS followed by in-depth diagnostic assessment [10]. In a Norwegian study, 33% of patients on opioid maintenance therapy [51] and in the Italian study, 19.4% [25] were positive for ADHD using the ASRS. Among patients with benzodiazepine dependence, 32% of them screened positive on ADHD [32].

Brazilian study validated the translated version of the adult self-report The Brown Attention-Deficit Disorder Scale (BADDS) using the ASRS as the gold standard [52], but ASRS appears to be more appropriate screener that BADDS in SUD patients [53]. Conners' Adult ADHD Diagnostic Interview for DSM-IV (CAADID) proved to be a diagnostic tool that can also be used during active substance use [54]. Study investigating the clinical utility of two self-report screening instruments such as Conners' Adult ADHD Rating Scale screening Self-Rating (CAARS-S-SR) and the ASRS in alcohol use disorder showed many false-negative results (ASRS: 89.5%; CAARS-S-SR: 92.3%) which indicates underreporting of ADHD symptoms. Authors suggested that underreporting of ADHD symptoms in ASRS and CAARS-S-SR of alcohol use disorder patients requires lower cut-off values to detect the majority of ADHD [55].

In a recent study from international multi-center, the Mini-International Neuropsychiatric Interview (MINI-Plus) on patients with substance use disorders was validated for the screening of adult ADHD in treatment-seeking SUD patients [56]. Another tool in understanding the possible causes and motivations behind substance misuse and its dependency is Substance Transitions in Addiction Rating Scale (STARS) where the subscales produced meaningful and reliable factors that supported the self-medication and behavioral disinhibition hypotheses of substance use motivation [36].

3.4 Treatment

Comorbid ADHD and SUD represent a challenge for health-care providers as the pharmacological trials have found mix results for efficacy [8]. The reviews on ADHD medications for ADHD with SUD point out limited efficacy of treatment, but more recent trials using psychostimulants in robust dosing have demonstrated positive results [57–60].

Guidelines recommend that when ADHD coexists with other psychopathologies in adults, the most impairing condition should generally be treated first [58]. Another approach is to first achieve abstinence before treating ADHD, where the main goal is to reduce the risk of diversion of stimulant medication [57]. The international consensus statement recommends long-acting stimulant medication [10].

While previous concerns arose whether stimulant therapy would increase the ultimate risk for substance abuse, recent studies have indicated that pharmacologic treatment appears to reduce the risk of substance abuse in individuals with ADHD [61]. Findings from 19 large open studies and controlled clinical trials show that the use of atomoxetine or extended-release methylphenidate formulations, together with psychological therapy, yield promising though inconclusive results about short-term efficacy of these drugs in the treatment of adult ADHD in patients with SUD and no other severe mental disorders. However, the efficacy of these drugs is scant or lacking in treating concurrent SUD [62]. The concern is as indicated by American study that ADHD is prevalent among chronic methamphetamine users, who are at increased risk for persistence of childhood diagnoses of ADHD into their adult years. ADHD also appears to play an important role in methamphetamine-associated disability, indicating that targeted ADHD screening and treatment may help to improve real-world outcomes for individuals with methamphetamine use disorders [63].

A meta-analysis on the efficacy of atomoxetine in treating adult ADHD showed atomoxetine is efficacious in treating adult ADHD compared to placebo, though the efficacy is significantly superior for inattention than hyperactivity/impulsivity [64]. Study on alcohol-dependent patients with and without a diagnosis of ADHD hypothesized that atomoxetine could reduce the impulsivity trait [65]. A small study reported that atomoxetine may improve some ADHD symptoms but does not reduce marijuana use in marijuana-dependent adults with ADHD [66].

A small study on ADHD patient with cocaine use disorder showed that behaviors reflecting cocaine addiction were sharply reduced during the stimulant treatment of adult ADHD, and were not correlated with age, gender, familiarity, length of treatment, or medication used. Cocaine use disorder improvement was closely correlated with adult ADHD improvement [67]. Earlier data show that patients with ADHD and comorbid cocaine dependence do not benefit significantly from treatment with methylphenidate, where Dutch study showed that low dopamine transporter occupancy is not the reason for that. Authors also suggest that higher dosages of methylphenidate in these patients are probably not the solution and that medications directed at other pharmacological targets should be considered in these comorbid ADHD patients [68]. ADHD patients with cocaine dependence are a distinctly more impulsive subpopulation compared to ADHD patients without cocaine dependence on objective measures of impulsivity. These findings are relevant for optimizing psycho-education and treatment of ADHD patients with comorbid SUD [41].

Sweden placebo-controlled double-blind study reported that methylphenidate treatment reduces ADHD symptoms and the risk for relapse to substance use in criminal offenders with ADHD and substance dependence [69]. Norway study reported about the safety and utility of central stimulant medications for patients with ADHD who are receiving opioid maintenance treatment [70]. Sustained-release methylphenidate in a double-blind, placebo-controlled trial for the treatment of ADHD in amphetamine abusers found no difference with regards to the craving for amphetamine or in retention in treatment [71]. Another double-blind, placebo-controlled study in adults with ADHD reported that extended-release methylphenidate was statistically superior to placebo in reducing emotional symptoms and a decline of obsessive-compulsive symptoms and those of problems with self-concept. Symptoms of anxiety, depression, anger and hostility, phobia, paranoid ideations and psychoticism were not improved [72]. A study that examined if stimulants would decrease marijuana use in a randomized controlled trial of extended-release mixed amphetamine salts for the treatment of co-occurring ADHD and cocaine use disorders found no significant baseline differences in marijuana use frequency and quantity [73].

A recent Dutch randomized clinical trial among SUD and ADHD patients reported that integrated cognitive behavioral therapy resulted in a significant improvement in ADHD symptoms in comorbid SUD and ADHD patients [74]. This finding leads to the conclusion that nonpharmacological interventions can contribute to ADHD symptom reduction in patients with comorbid ADHD and SUD. ADHD and SUD experts recommend that simultaneous and integrated treatment of ADHD and SUD, using a combination of pharmaco- and psychotherapy, is effective [10].

4. Conclusions

ADHD is highly comorbid with SUD, being diagnosed up to 20% in SUD patients. ADHD and SUD are believed to have shared pathophysiology. ADHD is associated with the majority of dependence diagnoses. A most used screening questionnaire for screening ADHD patients presenting with SUD is the ASRS. Evidence on pharmacological treatment is limited, but new trials support the use of a higher dose of long-acting stimulants as also recommended with a combination of psychotherapy by expert opinion. Finally, the decision to treat adult ADHD in the context of SUD depends on various factors, so clinical decisions should be individualized and based on a careful analysis of the advantages and disadvantages of pharmacological treatment for ADHD in the context of SUD. Given the prevalence of both ADHD and SUD, more research is needed to understand the theoretical and clinical implications of this comorbidity.

Conflict of interest

The authors declare no conflict of interest.

Author details

Anja Plemenitaš Ilješ
Department of Psychiatry, University Clinical Centre Maribor, Maribor, Slovenia

*Address all correspondence to: anja.plemenitas@ukc-mb.si

References

[1] American Psychiatric Association. Diagnostic and Statistical Manual of Mental Disorders. 5th ed. Arlington, VA: American Psychiatric Publishing; 2013

[2] Rowland AS, Skipper BJ, Umbach DM, Rabiner DL, Campbell RA, Naftel AJ, et al. The prevalence of ADHD in a population-based sample. Journal of Attention Disorders. 2015;**19**(9):741-754. DOI: 10.1177/1087054713513799

[3] Klein RG, Mannuzza S, Olazagasti MA, Roizen E, Hutchison JA, Lashua EC, et al. Clinical and functional outcome of childhood attention-deficit/hyperactivity disorder 33 years later. Archives of General Psychiatry. 2012;**69**(12):1295-1303. DOI: 10.1001/archgenpsychiatry.2012.271

[4] Faraone SV, Biederman J, Mick E. The age-dependent decline of attention deficit hyperactivity disorder: A meta-analysis of follow-up studies. Psychological Medicine. 2006;**36**(2):159-165. DOI: 10.1017/S003329170500471X

[5] Slobodin O, Davidovitch M. Gender differences in objective and subjective measures of ADHD among clinic-referred children. Frontiers in Human Neuroscience. 2019;**13**:441. DOI: 10.3389/fnhum.2019.00441

[6] Tripp G, Wickens JR. Neurobiology of ADHD. Neuropharmacology. 2009;**57**(7-8):579-589. DOI: 10.1016/j.neuropharm.2009.07.026

[7] Koob GF, Volkow ND. Neurocircuitry of addiction. Neuropsychopharmacology. 2010;**35**(1):217-238. DOI: 10.1038/npp.2009.110

[8] van der Burg D, Crunelle CL, Matthys F, van den Brink W. Diagnosis and treatment of patients with comorbid substance use disorder and adult attention-deficit and hyperactivity disorder: A review of recent publications. Current Opinion in Psychiatry. 2019;**32**(4):300-306. DOI: 10.1097/YCO.0000000000000513

[9] van Emmerik-van Oortmerssen K, van de Glind G, van den Brink W, Smit F, Crunelle CL, Swets M, et al. Prevalence of attention-deficit hyperactivity disorder in substance use disorder patients: A meta-analysis and meta-regression analysis. Drug and Alcohol Dependence. 2012;**122**(1-2):11-19. DOI: 10.1016/j.drugalcdep.2011.12.007

[10] Crunelle CL, van den Brink W, Moggi F, Konstenius M, Franck J, Levin FR, et al. Group Ic, and Matthys F. international consensus statement on screening, diagnosis and treatment of substance use disorder patients with comorbid attention deficit/hyperactivity disorder. European Addiction Research. 2018;**24**(1):43-51. DOI: 10.1159/000487767

[11] Konstenius M, Leifman A, van Emmerik-van Oortmerssen K, van de Glind G, Franck J, Moggi F, et al. Childhood trauma exposure in substance use disorder patients with and without ADHD. Addictive Behaviors. 2017;**65**:118-124. 10.1016/j.addbeh.2016.10.016

[12] Yule AM, Martelon M, Faraone SV, Carrellas N, Wilens TE, Biederman J. Examining the association between attention deficit hyperactivity disorder and substance use disorders: A familial risk analysis. Journal of Psychiatric Research. 2017;**85**:49-55. DOI: 10.1016/j.jpsychires.2016.10.018

[13] Walters RK, Polimanti R, Johnson EC, McClintick JN, Adams MJ, Adkins AE, et al. Transancestral GWAS of alcohol dependence reveals common genetic underpinnings with psychiatric disorders.

Nature Neuroscience. 2018;**21**(12):1656-1669. DOI: 10.1038/s41593-018-0275-1

[14] Gurriarán X, Rodríguez-López J, Flórez G, Pereiro C, Fernández JM, Fariñas E, et al. Relationships between substance abuse/dependence and psychiatric disorders based on polygenic scores. Genes, Brain and Behavior. 2019;**18**(3):e12504. DOI: 10.1111/gbb.12504

[15] Carpentier PJ, Arias Vasquez A, Hoogman M, Onnink M, Kan CC, Kooij JJ, et al. Shared and unique genetic contributions to attention deficit/hyperactivity disorder and substance use disorders: A pilot study of six candidate genes. European Neuropsychopharmacology. 2013;**23**(6):448-457. DOI: 10.1016/j.euroneuro.2012.07.003

[16] Groenman AP, Greven CU, van Donkelaar MM, Schellekens A, van Hulzen KJ, Rommelse N, et al. Dopamine and serotonin genetic risk scores predicting substance and nicotine use in attention deficit/hyperactivity disorder. Addiction Biology. 2016;**21**(4):915-923. DOI: 10.1111/adb.12230

[17] Coppola M, Sacchetto G, Mondola R. Craving for heroin: Difference between methadone maintenance therapy patients with and without ADHD. Trends in Psychiatry and Psychotherapy. 2019;**41**(1):83-86. DOI: 10.1590/2237-6089-2017-0159

[18] Quinn PD, Chang Z, Hur K, Gibbons RD, Lahey BB, Rickert ME, et al. ADHD medication and substance-related problems. The American Journal of Psychiatry. 2017;**174**(9):877-885. DOI: 10.1176/appi.ajp.2017.16060686

[19] van de Glind G, Konstenius M, MWJ K, van Emmerik-van Oortmerssen K, Carpentier PJ, Kaye S, et al. Variability in the prevalence of adult ADHD in treatment seeking substance use disorder patients: Results from an international multi-center study exploring DSM-IV and DSM-5 criteria. Genes, Brain, and Behavior. 2014;**134**:158-166. DOI: 10.1111/gbb.12504

[20] Luderer M, Sick C, Kaplan-Wickel N, Reinhard I, Richter A, Kiefer F, et al. Prevalence estimates of ADHD in a sample of inpatients with alcohol dependence. Journal of Attention Disorders. 2018:1087054717750272. DOI: 10.1177/1087054717750272

[21] Umar MU, Salihu AS, Owolabi SD. Prevalence and correlates of ADHD in individuals with substance use disorder in Nigeria. ADHD Attention Deficit and Hyperactivity Disorders. 2017;**9**(3):189-198. DOI: 10.1007/s12402-017-0218-9

[22] Kaye S, Darke S, Torok M. Attention deficit hyperactivity disorder (ADHD) among illicit psychostimulant users: A hidden disorder? Addiction. 2013;**108**(5):923-931. DOI: 10.1016/j.psychres.2017.01.052

[23] Delavenne H, Ballon N, Charles-Nicolas A, Garcia FD, Thibaut F, Lacoste J. Attention deficit hyperactivity disorder is associated with a more severe pattern of cocaine consumption in cocaine users from French West Indies. Journal of Addiction Medicine. 2011;**5**(4):284-288. DOI: 10.1097/ADM.0b013e31821b4038

[24] Daigre C, Roncero C, Grau-Lopez L, Martinez-Luna N, Prat G, Valero S, et al. Attention deficit hyperactivity disorder in cocaine-dependent adults: A psychiatric comorbidity analysis. The American Journal on Addictions. 2013;**22**(5):466-473. DOI: 10.1111/j.1521-0391.2013.12047.x

[25] Lugoboni F, Levin FR, Pieri MC, Manfredini M, Zamboni L, Somaini L, et al. Co-occurring attention deficit

hyperactivity disorder symptoms in adults affected by heroin dependence: Patients characteristics and treatment needs. Psychiatry Research. 2017;**250**:210-216. DOI: 10.1111/dar.12249

[26] Carpentier PJ, van Gogh MT, Knapen LJ, Buitelaar JK, De Jong CA. Influence of attention deficit hyperactivity disorder and conduct disorder on opioid dependence severity and psychiatric comorbidity in chronic methadone-maintained patients. European Addiction Research. 2011;**17**(1):10-20. DOI: 10.1159/000321259

[27] Tejeda-Romero C, Kobashi-Margáin RA, Alvarez-Arellano L, Corona JC, González-García N. Differences in substance use, psychiatric disorders and social factors between Mexican adolescents and young adults. American Journal on Addictions. 2018;**27**(8):625-631. DOI: 10.1111/ajad.12808

[28] De Alwis D, Lynskey MT, Reiersen AM, Agrawal A. Attention-deficit/hyperactivity disorder subtypes and substance use and use disorders in NESARC. Addictive Behaviors. 2014;**39**(8):1278-1285. DOI: 10.1016/j.addbeh.2014.04.003

[29] Ameringer KJ, Leventhal AM. Associations between attention deficit hyperactivity disorder symptom domains and DSM-IV lifetime substance dependence. The American Journal on Addictions. 2013;**22**(1):23-32. DOI: 10.1111/j.1521-0391.2013.00325.x

[30] Levy S, Katusic SK, Colligan RC, Weaver AL, Killian JM, Voigt RG, et al. Childhood ADHD and risk for substance dependence in adulthood: A longitudinal, population-based study. PLoS One. 2014;**9**(8):e105640. DOI: 10.1371/journal.pone.0105640

[31] Ilbegi S, Groenman AP, Schellekens A, Hartman CA, Hoekstra PJ, Franke B, et al. Substance use and nicotine dependence in persistent, remittent, and late-onset ADHD: A 10-year longitudinal study from childhood to young adulthood. Journal of Neurodevelopmental Disorders. 2018;**10**(1):42. DOI: 10.1186/s11689-018-9260-y

[32] Tamburin S, Federico A, Morbioli L, Faccini M, Casari R, Zamboni L, et al. Screening for adult attention deficit/hyperactivity disorder in high-dose benzodiazepine dependent patients. The American Journal on Addictions. 2017;**26**(6):610-614. DOI: 10.1111/ajad.12573

[33] Fatséas M, Hurmic H, Serre F, Debrabant R, Daulouède JP, Denis C, et al. Addiction severity pattern associated with adult and childhood attention deficit hyperactivity disorder (ADHD) in patients with addictions. Psychiatry Research. 2016;**246**:656-662. DOI: 10.1016/j.psychres.2016.10.071

[34] Torok M, Darke S, Kaye S. Attention deficit hyperactivity disorder and severity of substance use: The role of comorbid psychopathology. Psychology of Addictive Behaviors. 2012;**26**(4): 974-979. DOI: 10.1037/a0027846

[35] Carpentier PJ, Knapen LJ, van Gogh MT, Buitelaar JK, De Jong CA. Addiction in developmental perspective: Influence of conduct disorder severity, subtype, and attention-deficit hyperactivity disorder on problem severity and comorbidity in adults with opioid dependence. Journal of Addictive Diseases. 2012;**31**(1):45-59. DOI: 10.1080/10550887.2011.642756

[36] Young S, Gonzalez RA, Wolff K, Mutch L, Malet-Lambert I, Gudjonsson GH. Transitions and motivations for substance misuse in prison inmates with ADHD and conduct disorder: Validation of a new instrument. Journal of Dual

Diagnosis. 2017;**13**(2):91-100. DOI: 10.1080/15504263.2017.1290859

[37] Camargo CH, Dornelles TF, Barszcz K, Martins EA. Attention deficit hyperactivity disorder and drug addiction rehabilitation patients. Arquivos de Neuro-Psiquiatria. 2016;**74**(12):1003-1007. DOI: 10.1590/0004-282x20160163

[38] Breyer JL, Lee S, Winters KC, August GJ, Realmuto GM. A longitudinal study of childhood ADHD and substance dependence disorders in early adulthood. The American Journal on Addictions. 2014;**28**(1):238-246. DOI: 10.1111/ajad.12808

[39] Young JT, Carruthers S, Kaye S, Allsop S, Gilsenan J, Degenhardt L, et al. Comorbid attention deficit hyperactivity disorder and substance use disorder complexity and chronicity in treatment-seeking adults. Drug and Alcohol Review. 2015;**34**(6):683-693. DOI: 10.1080/15504263.2017.1290859

[40] Daurio AM, Aston SA, Schwandt ML, Bukhari MO, Bouhlal S, Farokhnia M, et al. Impulsive personality traits mediate the relationship between adult attention-deficit/hyperactivity symptoms and alcohol dependence severity. Alcoholism, Clinical and Experimental Research. 2018;**42**(1):173-183. DOI: 10.1111/acer.13538

[41] Crunelle CL, Veltman DJ, van Emmerik-van Oortmerssen K, Booij J, van den Brink W. Impulsivity in adult ADHD patients with and without cocaine dependence. Drug and Alcohol Dependence. 2013;**129**(1-2):18-24. DOI: 10.1016/j.drugalcdep.2012.09.006

[42] Stevens L, Roeyers H, Dom G, Joos L, Vanderplasschen W. Impulsivity in cocaine-dependent individuals with and without attention-deficit/hyperactivity disorder. European Addiction Research. 2015;**21**(3):131-143. DOI: 10.1159/000369008

[43] Miguel CS, Martins PA, Moleda N, Klein M, Chaim-Avancini T, Gobbo MA, et al. Cognition and impulsivity in adults with attention deficit hyperactivity disorder with and without cocaine and/or crack dependence. Drug and Alcohol Dependence. 2016;**160**:97-104. DOI: 10.1016/j.drugalcdep.2015.12.040

[44] Vergara-Moragues E, Gonzalez-Saiz F, Lozano Rojas O, Bilbao Acedos I, Fernandez Calderon F, Betanzos Espinosa P, et al. Diagnosing adult attention deficit/hyperactivity disorder in patients with cocaine dependence: Discriminant validity of Barkley executive dysfunction symptoms. European Addiction Research. 2011;**17**(6):279-284. DOI: 10.1159/000329725

[45] Seitz A, Wapp M, Burren Y, Stutz S, Schläfli K, Moggi F. Association between craving and attention deficit/hyperactivity disorder symptoms among patients with alcohol use disorders. The American Journal on Addictions. 2013;**22**(3):292-296. DOI: 10.1111/j.1521-0391.2012.12000.x

[46] Bacskai E, Czobor P, Gerevich J. Trait aggression, depression and suicidal behavior in drug dependent patients with and without ADHD symptoms. Psychiatry Research. 2012;**200**(2-3):719-723. DOI: 10.1016/j.psychres.2012.06.005

[47] Young S, Wells J, Gudjonsson GH. Predictors of offending among prisoners: The role of attention-deficit hyperactivity disorder and substance use. Journal of Psychopharmacology. 2011;**25**(11):1524-1532. DOI: 10.1177/0269881110370502

[48] Liao YT, Chen CY, Ng MH, Huang KY, Shao WC, Lin TY, et al. Depression and severity of substance dependence among heroin dependent patients with ADHD symptoms. The American Journal on Addictions.

2017;**26**(1):26-33. DOI: 10.1111/ajad.12487

[49] Peles E, Schreiber S, Sutzman A, Adelson M. Attention deficit hyperactivity disorder and obsessive-compulsive disorder among former heroin addicts currently in methadone maintenance treatment. Psychopathology. 2012;**45**(5):327-333. DOI: 10.1159/000336219

[50] Kooij J, Francken M. Diagnostic Interview for ADHD in Adults (DIVA). The Hague: DIVA Foundation; 2010

[51] Fiksdal Abel K, Ravndal E, Clausen T, Bramness JG. Attention deficit hyperactivity disorder symptoms are common in patients in opioid maintenance treatment. European Addiction Research. 2017;**23**(6):298-305. DOI: 10.1159/000484240

[52] Kakubo SM, Mendez M, Silveira JD, Maringolo L, Nitta C, Silveira DXD, et al. Translation and validation of the Brown attention-deficit disorder scale for use in Brazil: Identifying cases of attention-deficit/hyperactivity disorder among samples of substance users and non-users. Cross-cultural validation study. São Paulo Medical Journal. 2018;**136**(2):157-164. DOI: 10.1590/1516-3180.2017.0227121217

[53] van de Glind G, van den Brink W, Koeter MW, Carpentier PJ, van Emmerik-van Oortmerssen K, Kaye S, et al. Validity of the adult ADHD self-report scale (ASRS) as a screener for adult ADHD in treatment seeking substance use disorder patients. Drug and Alcohol Dependence. 2013;**132**(3):587-596. DOI: 10.1016/j.drugalcdep.2013.04.010

[54] van Emmerik-van Oortmerssen K, Vedel E, Kramer FJ, Koeter MW, Schoevers RA, van den Brink W. Diagnosing ADHD during active substance use: Feasible or flawed? Drug and Alcohol Dependence. 2017;**180**:371-375. DOI: 10.1016/j.drugalcdep.2017.07.039

[55] Luderer M, Kaplan-Wickel N, Richter A, Reinhard I, Kiefer F, Weber T. Screening for adult attention-deficit/hyperactivity disorder in alcohol dependent patients: Underreporting of ADHD symptoms in self-report scales. Drug and Alcohol Dependence. 2019;**195**:52-58. DOI: 10.1016/j.drugalcdep.2018.11.020

[56] Palma-Alvarez RF, Barta C, Carpentier PJ, Carruthers S, Crunelle CL, Demetrovics Z, et al. Validity of the ADHD module of the mini international neuropsychiatric interview PLUS for screening of adult ADHD in treatment seeking substance use disorder patients: ADHD screening with MINI-Plus. Revista de Psiquiatría y Salud Mental. 2020. DOI: 10.1016/j.rpsm.2020.04.013

[57] Dirks H, Scherbaum N, Kis B, Mette C. ADHD in adults and comorbid substance use disorder: Prevalence, clinical diagnostics and integrated therapy. Fortschritte der Neurologie-Psychiatrie. 2017;**85**(6):336-344. DOI: 10.1055/s-0043-100763

[58] Katzman MA, Bilkey TS, Chokka PR, Fallu A, Klassen LJ. Adult ADHD and comorbid disorders: Clinical implications of a dimensional approach. BMC Psychiatry. 2017;**17**(1):302. DOI: 10.1186/s12888-017-1463-3

[59] Carpentier PJ, Levin FR. Pharmacological treatment of ADHD in addicted patients: What does the literature tell us? Harvard Review of Psychiatry. 2017;**25**(2):50-64. DOI: 10.1097/HRP.0000000000000122

[60] Cook J, Lloyd-Jones M, Arunogiri S, Ogden E, Bonomo Y. Managing attention deficit hyperactivity disorder in adults using illicit

psychostimulants: A systematic review. The Australian and New Zealand Journal of Psychiatry. 2017;**51**(9):876-885. DOI: 10.1177/0004867417714878

[61] Wilens TE. Impact of ADHD and its treatment on substance abuse in adults. The Journal of Clinical Psychiatry. 2004;**65**(Suppl 3):38-45

[62] Perez de los Cobos J, Sinol N, Perez V, Trujols J. Pharmacological and clinical dilemmas of prescribing in co-morbid adult attention-deficit/hyperactivity disorder and addiction. British Journal of Clinical Pharmacology. 2014;**77**(2):337-356. DOI: 10.1111/bcp.12045

[63] Obermeit LC, Cattie JE, Bolden KA, Marquine MJ, Morgan EE, Franklin DR Jr, et al. Attention-deficit/hyperactivity disorder among chronic methamphetamine users: Frequency, persistence, and adverse effects on everyday functioning. Addictive Behaviors. 2013;**38**(12):2874-2878. DOI: 10.1016/j.addbeh.2013.08.010

[64] Ravishankar V, Chowdappa SV, Benegal V, Muralidharan K. The efficacy of atomoxetine in treating adult attention deficit hyperactivity disorder (ADHD): A meta-analysis of controlled trials. Asian Journal of Psychiatry. 2016;**24**:53-58. DOI: 10.1016/j.ajp.2016.08.017

[65] Coppola M, Mondola R. Impulsivity in alcohol-dependent patients with and without ADHD: The role of atomoxetine. Journal of Psychoactive Drugs. 2018;**50**(4):361-366. DOI: 10.1080/02791072.2018.1471247

[66] McRae-Clark AL, Carter RE, Killeen TK, Carpenter MJ, White KG, Brady KT. A placebo-controlled trial of atomoxetine in marijuana-dependent individuals with attention deficit hyperactivity disorder. The American Journal on Addictions. 2010;**19**(6):481-489. DOI: 10.1111/j.1521-0391.2010.00076.x

[67] Manni C, Cipollone G, Pallucchini A, Maremmani AGI, Perugi G, Maremmani I. Remarkable reduction of cocaine use in dual disorder (adult attention deficit hyperactive disorder/cocaine use disorder) patients treated with medications for ADHD. International Journal of Environmental Research and Public Health. 2019;**16**(20). DOI: 10.3390/ijerph16203911

[68] Crunelle CL, van den Brink W, Veltman DJ, van Emmerik-van Oortmerssen K, Dom G, Schoevers RA, et al. Low dopamine transporter occupancy by methylphenidate as a possible reason for reduced treatment effectiveness in ADHD patients with cocaine dependence. European Neuropsychopharmacology. 2013;**23**(12):1714-1723. DOI: 10.1016/j.euroneuro.2013.05.002

[69] Konstenius M, Jayaram-Lindström N, Guterstam J, Beck O, Philips B, Franck J. Methylphenidate for attention deficit hyperactivity disorder and drug relapse in criminal offenders with substance dependence: A 24-week randomized placebo-controlled trial. Addiction. 2014;**109**(3):440-449. DOI: 10.1111/add.12369

[70] Abel KF, Bramness JG, Martinsen EW. Stimulant medication for ADHD in opioid maintenance treatment. Journal of Dual Diagnosis. 2014;**10**(1):32-38. DOI: 10.1080/15504263.2013.867657

[71] Konstenius M, Jayaram-Lindstrom N, Beck O, Franck J. Sustained release methylphenidate for the treatment of ADHD in amphetamine abusers: A pilot study. Drug and Alcohol Dependence. 2010;**108**(1-2):130-133. DOI: 10.1016/j.drugalcdep.2009.11.006

[72] Rosler M, Retz W, Fischer R, Ose C, Alm B, Deckert J, et al.

Twenty-four-week treatment with extended release methylphenidate improves emotional symptoms in adult ADHD. The World Journal of Biological Psychiatry. 2010;**11**(5):709-718. DOI: 10.3109/15622971003624197

[73] Notzon DP, Mariani JJ, Pavlicova M, Glass A, Mahony AL, Brooks DJ, et al. Mixed-amphetamine salts increase abstinence from marijuana in patients with co-occurring attention-deficit/ hyperactivity disorder and cocaine dependence. The American Journal on Addictions. 2016;**25**(8):666-672. DOI: 10.1111/ajad.12467

[74] van Emmerik-van Oortmerssen K, Vedel E, Kramer FJ, Blankers M, Dekker JJM, van den Brink W, et al. Integrated cognitive behavioral therapy for ADHD in adult substance use disorder patients: Results of a randomized clinical trial. Drug and Alcohol Dependence. 2019;**197**:28-36. DOI: 10.1016/j.drugalcdep.2018.12.023